Handbook of Nephrology

Handbook of Nephrology

SECOND EDITION

Peter E. Gower BSc, MD, FRCP
Consultant Physician
Charing Cross Hospital
London

OXFORD

BLACKWELL SCIENTIFIC PUBLICATIONS

LONDON EDINBURGH BOSTON

MELBOURNE PARIS BERLIN VIENNA

© 1983, 1991 by
Blackwell Scientific Publications
Editorial Offices:
Osney Mead, Oxford OX2 0EL
25 John Street, London WC1N 2BL
23 Ainslie Place, Edinburgh EH3 6AJ
3 Cambridge Center, Cambridge
    Massachusetts 02142, USA
54 University Street, Carlton
    Victoria 3053, Australia

Other Editorial Offices:
Arnette SA
2, rue Casimir-Delavigne
75006 Paris
France

Blackwell Wissenschaft
Meinekestrasse 4
D-1000 Berlin 15
Germany

Blackwell MZV
Feldgasse 13
A-1238 Wien
Austria

First published 1983
(Under the title *Nephrology Pocket
Consultant*)
Spanish edition 1986
Second edition 1991

Set by Setrite Typesetters, Hong Kong
Printed and bound in Great Britain at
The Alden Press, Oxford.

DISTRIBUTORS

    Marston Book Services Ltd
    PO Box 87
    Oxford OX2 0DT
    (*Orders*: Tel: 0865 791155
             Fax: 0865 791927
             Telex: 837515)

USA
    Mosby-Year Book, Inc.
    11830 Westline Industrial Drive
    St Louis, Missouri 63146
    (*Orders*: Tel: 800 633−6699)

Canada
    Mosby-Year Book, Inc.
    5240 Finch Avenue East
    Scarborough, Ontario
    (*Orders*: Tel: 416 298−1588)

Australia
    Blackwell Scientific Publications
    (Australia) Pty Ltd
    54 University Street
    Carlton, Victoria 3053
    (*Orders*: Tel: 03 347−0300)

British Library
Cataloguing in Publication Data
Gower, P.E.
    Handbook of nephrology − 2nd ed.
    1. Man. Kidneys. Diseases
    I. Title
    616.61

    ISBN 0−632−02164−0

Contents

Preface to the second edition

A number of important changes in nephrological practice have taken place since the first edition was published, particularly in the management of acute renal failure, chronic renal failure, dialysis and transplantation. These changes are reflected in large parts of the book, where many topics have been rewritten, as well as numerous minor alterations in other chapters.

Preface to the first edition

The practice of nephrology has grown apace and junior medical staff may be confronted with a variety of new medical and technical problems in this field. This book is intended to help decision-making in common clinical situations in adult patients with renal disease. It is not a textbook, and discussion of controversial topics is kept to a minimum.

It is hoped the book will also prove of value to undergraduate students, as well as nurses and technical staff who work in renal units and promote the practice of nephrology, so that our patients will benefit.

Acknowledgements

I am grateful to the following for their help in preparing this book: Professor J.S. Cameron for permission to reproduce the figure on p. 91 (1979: The natural history of glomerulo-nephritis. In Black, Sir Douglas A.K. and Jones, N.F. (eds) *Renal Disease*, 4th ed. p. 370. Oxford, Blackwell Scientific Publications); Drs R.S. Walton and O.L.M. Bijvoet for the phosphate threshold nomogram (1975: *Lancet* **ii**, 309); Dr D. Woodrow for the photomicrographs; Mr M. Duffy, Miss M. Hudson and Mrs J. Brown of the Department of Medical Illustration, Charing Cross Hospital Medical School, for all the figures; and Mrs J. Howard, District Dietitian, Charing Cross Hospital, for the diet sheets.

I am indebted to Drs Pat Parfrey and David Saltissi for their constructive comments, Mrs S. Burke for her skills in typing the manuscript, and my wife, Pearl, for her tolerance during the preparation of the book.

1: Applied anatomy

1.1 Gross anatomy

The kidneys lie obliquely in the paravertebral gutters, the right slightly lower than the left. Posteriorly, they are related above the 12th rib to the pleura and the diaphragm and below, by the paravertebral muscles (Fig. 1.1). Anteriorly lie the spleen, stomach, pancreas and jejunum on the left, the liver, colon and duodenum on the right (Fig. 1.2). The kidneys measure approximately 12–14 cm (the length of 3 lumbar vertebral bodies) and in the adult should not vary by more than 1.5 cm in length. In the erect position the right kidney is often very mobile but this has no known pathological significance.

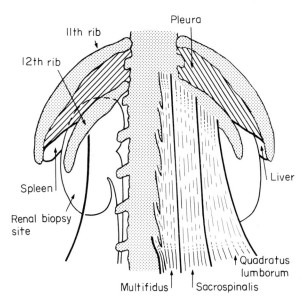

Fig. 1.1 Posterior relations of the kidney.

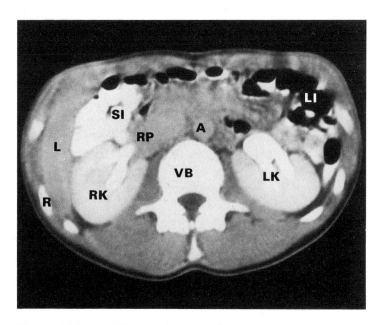

Fig. 1.2 Abdominal CT scan at level L3. R: rib; SI: small intestine; LI: large intestine; A: aorta; RP: renal pedicle; RK: right kidney; LK: left kidney; and VB: vertebral body.

1.2 Internal architecture

The following points can be noted on Figure 1.3:

1 The renal outline is smooth and should be visible on urograms especially if tomograms are undertaken.

2 A line joining the tip of the papillae runs parallel with the renal outline, apart from the upper and lower poles where the renal substance is expanded.

3 The kidney is made up of a series of lobules which extend from one renal column to the next. Persistence of fetal lobulation occasionally occurs in adult life.

4 The number of papillae and corresponding calyces varies from approximately 6–8 to as many as 20. The upper and lower pole calyces tend to be compound (contain several minor calyces draining into one major calyx).

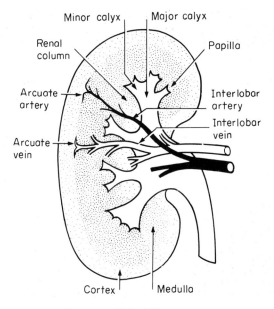

Fig. 1.3 Internal architecture of the kidney.

5 The renal arteries arise from the aorta just below the superior mesenteric artery. Multiple (2–4) arteries are not uncommon and may be difficult to visualize on aortography. Venous drainage is usually via a single vein to the inferior vena cava.

1.3 Anatomical variations

A large number of developmental abnormalities of varying clinical importance have been detected and include:
- supernumary kidneys
- solitary kidneys
- horseshoe kidney (Fig. 1.4)
- pelvic kidney (Fig. 1.5)
- crossed ectopia (Fig. 1.6)
- bifid systems: duplex kidney, duplex ureter, ectopic ureteric orifice (Fig. 1.7)
- bladder abnormalities, e.g. ureterocoele, ectopia vesicae

A *ureterocoele* is a minor abnormality of the intramural part of the ureter whereby a 'sleeve' of ureter is invaginated through

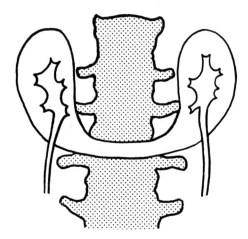

Fig. 1.4 Horseshoe kidney.

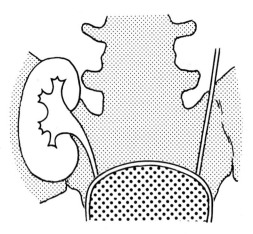

Fig. 1.5 Pelvic kidney.

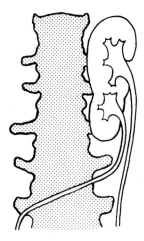

Fig. 1.6 Crossed ectopia.

the bladder mucosa. This minor abnormality is probably of no clinical significance.

Ectopia vesicae is a severe abnormality where there is absence of the lower anterior abdominal wall, part of the bladder and usually part of the symphysis pubis. Early reconstructive surgery is required to correct drainage abnormalities but most patients eventually need an ileal conduit.

Occasionally more than one congenital abnormality may co-exist, e.g. most ectopic kidneys show malrotation. Most of the abnormalities may be complicated by obstruction, stones and infection. Vesico-ureteric reflux may be associated with ectopic ureters. Note that ectopic ureters always follow a simple rule — the ureters draining the upper kidney moiety (if completely separate) pass below the ureter draining the lower kidney moiety and may empty below the bladder sphincter, causing incontinence, or into the vagina (Fig. 1.7). Retrocaval ureters occur only on the right side, and may be associated with obstruction to the kidney on that side.

All congenital abnormalities may be difficult to spot on urography, e.g. careful inspection of the bony pelvis may show

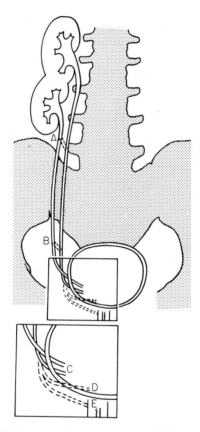

Fig. 1.7 Duplex kidney and ureters. A and B: possible joining sites of the ureters; C: anatomical relation of the duplex ureters draining separately; and D and E: possible sites of ectopic ureters (D: below bladder neck; E: into the vagina).

a pelvic kidney in a patient who has apparently only one kidney.

1.4 Microscopical anatomy

Each kidney contains approximately 1 million nephrons, each nephron consisting of a glomerulus, proximal convoluted tubule, loop of Henle, and distal convoluted tubules leading to a collecting duct (Fig. 1.8). There are two subdivisions of the

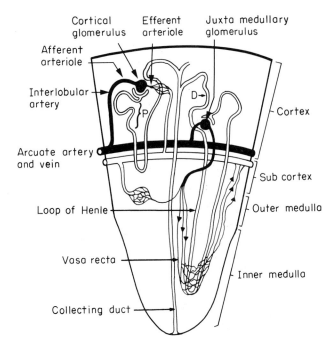

Fig. 1.8 Internal renal architecture. P: proximal convoluted tubule; and D: distal convoluted tubule.

nephron: superficial (cortical) and deep (juxta medullary). The distal convoluted tubule passes between the afferent and efferent arterioles and the glomerulus to form the 'juxta glomerular apparatus'. Granules of renin have been found in the afferent arteriolar wall at this site and it is thought that baroreceptors in the arteriolar wall, sympathetic nerves and distal tubular sodium concentration all control renin release.

The afferent arteriole divides into glomerular capillaries (Fig. 1.9). The capillary loops are lined by a continuous layer of basement membrane (width 200–400 nm) supported by mesangial cells. The filtration barrier consists of fenestrated endothelial cell cytoplasm, basement membrane and foot processes (podocytes) of the epithelial cell. The barrier allows molecules of up to 50 000 mol.wt to pass with little restriction, albumin (mol.wt 60 000) is 10 000 times less filterable than

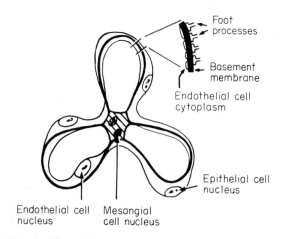

Fig. 1.9 Glomerular capillary wall and filtration barrier.

inulin; myeloperoxidase (mol.wt 160 000) and ferritin (mol.wt 480 000) are not filtered and are seen to be held up on the epithelial and endothelial sides of the basement membrane respectively. Filtration is determined not only by molecule size but also by shape and electrostatic charge. The mesangial cell acts not only as a supporting cell, but also has phagocytic and contractile properties.

1.5 Renal nerves and lymphatic drainage

The kidney is supplied by sympathetic fibres from T11 to L1 and by parasympathetic fibres from the vagus and pelvic splanchnic nerves. The nerves appear to supply the arteries and arterioles; a few reach the glomeruli. Lymphatic channels are also closely applied to arterioles and arteries and accompany the main renal vessels to the para-aortic nodes.

2: Investigation of renal function and structure

2.1 Renal blood flow, plasma flow and filtration fraction

The kidneys receive one-quarter of the cardiac output or approximately 1 litre of blood per minute in a normal adult. Assuming an haematocrit of 40%, the renal plasma flow (RPF) is 600 ml per minute. Since the glomerular filtration rate (GFR) is approximately 120 ml per minute, the fraction of plasma filtered (filtration fraction) is GFR/RPF or 0.20. Techniques for measuring renal blood flow include the Fick principle and the clearance of para-aminohippuric acid (PAH) or various isotopic techniques, and are largely experimental; the GFR is therefore used most commonly to assess kidney function. There are various drugs that will affect renal blood flow; some of which can be seen in Table 2.1.

Table 2.1 Drugs affecting renal blood flow.

Increase	Decrease
Dopamine	Adrenaline
Phenoxybenzamine	Noradrenaline
Vasodilators	β-blockers
Nadolol	Indomethacin
Captopril	
Frusemide	

2.2 Glomerular filtration rate

Creatinine clearance

Creatinine, an end-product of muscle metabolism, undergoes glomerular filtration and, in patients with normal renal function, is neither secreted nor reabsorbed by the tubule. It is, therefore, a convenient test of glomerular function. The 'clearance' of creatinine (or for that matter any substance handled by the kidney) represents the minimum volume of blood passing through the kidneys totally cleared of creatinine (or other substance) per unit time. Clearance of x is derived by knowing the concentration of x, in the urine U_x, the volume of urine passed V and concentration of x in the plasma P_x when clearance is $(U_x V)/P_x$. The calculation assumes that the concentration of x in blood and urine is constant for given time T. T for creatinine clearance is traditionally collected over 24 hours but shorter intervals may be used. It is important to note various factors.

1 The test depends on accurate urine collection.

2 Creatinine clearance should be corrected for body size and related to 1.73 m^2 (see Appendix 1).

3 In patients with advanced renal failure some creatinine is secreted by the tubules and creatinine clearance overestimates GFR by a small amount, and urea clearance underestimates GFR.

4 At lower rates of GFR ($\leq$15 ml per minute):

$$\text{GFR} = \frac{\text{Urea clearance} + \text{creatinine clearance}}{2}$$

^{51}Cr EDTA clearance

EDTA (ethylenediaminetetra-acetic acid) is excreted by glomerular filtration. This test has the advantage of not requiring any urine collection and is accurate. A dose of ^{51}Cr EDTA is given i.v. and serial samples (usually at 4 and 8 hours) are measured for isotopic activity. It has been shown that the decay curve is proportional to the GFR. One slight disadvantage is that, in patients with advanced renal failure, a 12-hour interval is required between blood sampling. The test is very useful for out-patients, children, and those with advanced renal failure.

Inulin clearance

Inulin clearance is an extremely accurate way of determining GFR but requires infusion pumps, possible catheterization and the difficult measurement of inulin in blood and urine. The test is reserved for research purposes only.

Level of plasma creatinine

There is an inverse exponential relation between creatinine clearance and plasma creatinine concentrations. For a GFR above 40 ml per minute, large changes in the creatinine clearance are accompanied by only slight changes in plasma creatinine. For example, a change in creatinine from 120 to 160 μmol/l may represent halving of renal function. In contrast, small changes in clearance below 40 ml per minute are associated with larger changes in plasma creatinine concentrations. In practice, therefore, the plasma creatinine has been used as an index of renal function, especially in patients with advanced renal failure. However, the plasma creatinine, like the clearance, is dependent on age, body size, and the muscle mass.

Derived creatinine clearance

It has been shown by Cockroft and Gault (1976: *Nephron* **16**, 31) that creatinine clearance may be predicted by using the following equation:

$$\text{GFR (ml per minute)} = \frac{1.23 \text{ (men) or } 1.04 \text{ (women)} \times (140\text{-age}) \times \text{weight (kg)}}{\text{plasma creatinine in } \mu\text{mol/l}}$$

This may be useful if 24-hour collections are difficult or if there is no access to a nuclear medicine laboratory. Limited experience has shown that this method underestimates GFR by about 10%.

Fractional clearance

Comparisons of a clearance of various substances, e.g. sodium, to that of creatinine, are widely used in experimental nephrology and are starting to be used in clinical practice. Since the urine volume is the same,

the fractional (percentage) clearance of sodium
= $(U/p$ sodium$)/(U/p$ creatinine$) \times 100$,
when U = urinary concentration and p = plasma
concentration.

Autoregulation

The kidney maintains a constant renal blood flow and GFR
over a wide range of perfusion pressure. The mechanisms
controlling this 'autoregulation' are ill-understood but involve
myogenic contractions in the afferent arteriole. Clinically, this
important regulating mechanism helps to control glomerular
filtration in states of both hypertension and hypotension.

2.3 Blood-urea and urea clearance

The blood-urea is a poor indicator of renal function, being
dependent on protein intake and catabolism of the patient.
Urea clearances do not reflect glomerular function since urea
is reabsorbed, and urea excretion depends also on urine flow
rates.

2.4 Tubular function

Proximal tubular function

Despite the fact that 80% of the tubular fluid, together with
most ions, amino acids and glucose, are reabsorbed by the
proximal tubule, tests of proximal tubular functions are difficult
and limited in application. Nevertheless, certain specific defects
of reabsorption may be detected, such as the reabsorption
capacity of glucose in renal glycosuria, phosphate in hyperparathyroidism and amino acids in cystinuria. There is a point
(threshold) at which maximum reabsorption occurs and beyond
which excretion takes place. Thresholds may be derived by
infusion experiments but it has been shown that it is possible
to use nomograms to measure phosphate threshold solely by
determining the concentration of phosphate and creatinine in

blood and urine (see Appendix 2). This may be very useful in the diagnosis of hyperparathyroidism.

Enzyme tests

The proximal tubular cells contain a variety of enzymes including N-acetyl-β-D-glucosaminidase (NAG). Urinary NAG concentration has been used as an index of proximal tubular damage but the test is non-specific since there are many ways of damaging kidney tubules other than by direct tubular toxicity. However, urinary NAG concentration may prove useful as an indicator of non-specific renal damage.

β_2-microglobulin

This has a mol.wt of about 11 800 and is normally found in blood and urine. β_2-microglobulin is reabsorbed by the proximal tubule. Determination of its clearance and comparison with albumin clearance, is a useful way of differentiating tubular from glomerular proteinuria, as an aid to the diagnosis of various tubular disorders (e.g. cadmium poisoning, Fanconi's syndrome, Balkan nephropathy).

As a guide:

$$\text{Tubular proteinuria} = \frac{U_{alb}}{U_{\beta_2 m}} \leqslant 15$$

$$\text{Glomular proteinuria} = \frac{U_{alb}}{U_{\beta_2 m}} \geqslant 1000$$

Other tubular function tests

Two tests are available clinically to measure distal tubular and collecting duct functions.

The ability to concentrate urine

Concentration of urine takes place in the medulla through the combined actions of the counter current system and the action of vasopressin on the collecting ducts. The concentrating ability of the kidney is determined by either water deprivation or the administration of vasopressin. Details of these investigations are given in Appendix 4.

In healthy people there is a wide variation in water excretion. Therefore, the concentration (osmolality) of the urine may vary from 50 to 1400 mmol/kg water. Whatever the urine flow, there is always a solute load to be cleared (osmolar clearance), which equals Uosm V/$p$osm. If urine and plasma osmolality are the same, osmolar clearance equals V. Usually, however, urine osmolality is either higher or lower than plasma osmolality and there is a volume of solute-free water to be added (positive free-water clearance C_{H_2O}) (when Uosm $>$ $p$osm) or subtracted (negative free-water clearance TC_{H_2O}) (when Uosm $<$ $p$osm) to the osmolar clearance. Free-water clearance is the volume of water needed to be added, or subtracted, from the urine to make the urine isosmotic with plasma:

$$C_{H_2O} = V - C\text{osm (hypotonic urine) ml/per minute;}$$

$$TC_{H_2O} = C\text{osm} - V \text{ (hypertonic urine) ml/per minute}$$

The concept of osmolar clearance is important in an understanding of disease states, notably diuretic use (p. 29), hepatorenal failure (p. 48) and, possible, cardiac failure.

Acidification of urine
Acidification of urine can take place in three ways.
1 Formation of H^+ ions for the exchange of bicarbonate in the proximal and distal tubule. H^+ ions are generated from H_2O and CO_2 in the tubular cell, by the action of carbonic anhydrase (CA). An increase in CO_2 results in an increase in HCO_3^- returned to the blood and excess H^+ ion excretion as titrable acidity (which is the amount of alkali in mmol required to titrate the urine to a pH of 7.4), and ammonia (Fig. 2.1).
2 Buffering of certain salts, including Na_2HPO_4, hydroxybutyrate and creatinine (Fig. 2.2).

Both 1 and 2 take place in all parts of the nephron but especially in the proximal tubule.
3 Formation of NH_4^+ ion. Ammonia is generated from glutamine in the tubular cells and combines with the H^+ ion to produce NH_4^+ ion. NH_4^+ diffuses poorly and is excreted in the urine. Note that ammonia diffuses in both directions, hence

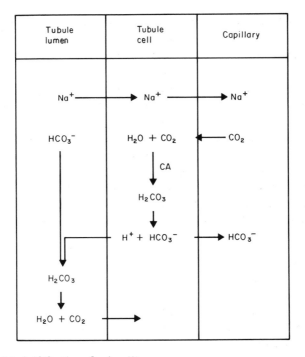

Fig. 2.1 Acidification of urine (1)

acidosis may be associated with NH_3 intoxication in patients with liver disease. Ammonia production takes place in all parts of the nephron but especially the distal tubule (Fig. 2.3).

In practice, the products of metabolism generate $50-100$ mmol of H^+ daily which is associated with a urinary pH of $\simeq 5.0$. Excess acid loads increase both the titrable acidity and ammonia excretion. The minimum pH of urine achieved is about 4.5. The ability of the kidney to excrete an acid load is undertaken using ammonium chloride (see Appendix 4), since NH_4Cl dissociates into NH_4 and Cl and the NH_4^+ is metabolized with CO_2 to produce H^+ ions:

$$2NH_4^+ + CO_2 \rightarrow CO(NH_2)_2 + H_2O + 2H^+$$

Disorders of urinary acidification occur with certain electrolyte deficiencies (e.g. hypokalaemia), renal tubular acidosis (p. 36) and are considered in greater detail in Chapter 3.

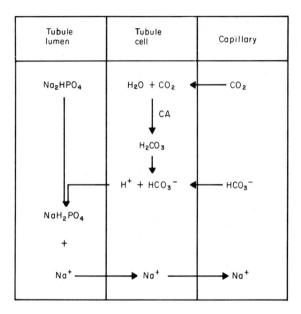

Fig. 2.2 Acidification of urine (2)

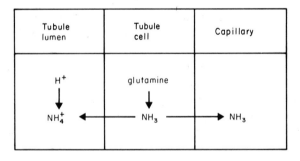

Fig. 2.3 Acidification of urine (3)

2.5 Radiological assessment

Intravenous urography (pyelography)

This remains the commonest test performed for assessing renal architecture. The following points must be borne in mind.

1 Absolute contraindication: known allergies to iodine.

2 Relative contraindication: diabetes with renal failure.

3 Special precautions: any patient with renal failure, especially those with salt and water overload and multiple myeloma. *Do not dehydrate or give laxatives to patients with renal failure.*

Modern contrast media contain either ionized iodine (e.g. Isopaque 370) for routine use or non-ionized iodine (e.g. Omnipaque 30) for use in patients with a history of previous reactions. Conventional preparations pre-urography include dehydration and purgation but good pictures may be obtained providing an adequate dose is used. Note that a high dose (2 ml/kg of body weight) is mandatory for patients with renal failure. There is no place for drip pyelography. Every urogram should be inspected during the procedure since special views, including oblique and prone films, as well as tomography, may be required. Early 1-minute films should be requested in renal artery stenosis and late, (4–6-hour) films in obstruction. Prone films show details of the ureters.

As with any X-ray, urograms need to be read methodically. Plain ('scout') films should be examined for bony abnormalities before scanning renal areas for size, stones or other soft-tissue abnormalities. The course of the ureters should be studied for stones and the bladder area for stones and soft-tissue abnormalities.

The 1-minute film should reveal outlines (nephrogram) and remaining renal films should show details of the pelvi-calyceal system (see Fig. 1.3). It is important to examine each calyx in turn, before looking at the ureters and bladder.

Details of the use of urograms are given in various sections throughout the book.

Antegrade pyelography

This is a very useful adjunct in the management of patients with suspected obstructive uropathy. Under screen control (or ultrasound), a fine-bore needle is introduced into the kidney pelvis or major calyx. Pressure studies are possible at this stage. Contrast material is injected to reveal the anatomy of the renal tract and likely site of obstruction. Finally, a 'pigtail' catheter can be introduced, on one side or both, into the renal pelvis to allow drainage, while other steps are taken to deal with the obstruction. This method is useful for transplant kidneys with suspected obstruction.

Angiography

Renal angiography may be undertaken either by direct arterial puncture (arteriography) or by digital subtraction angiography using the intravenous administration of contrast material. Either method shows the aorta and major renal vessels but details of intra-renal vessels are best shown by arteriography. Percutaneous angioplasty permits dilatation of renal arterial stenosis under direct vision. It is important to check the femoral artery cut-down site and peripheral pulses after the patient has returned to the ward.

Renal venography

A technique identical to that in arteriography is used to delineate the renal veins, e.g. to exclude thrombosis or for the measurement of the concentration of substances in the renal vein.

Ultrasound

Ultrasound has become one of the most useful techniques in the management of renal disorders. Resolution is of the order of 0.5 cm. Ultrasound is particularly useful for defining the length and depth of the kidney, diagnosing hydronephrosis and cystic lesions, and assisting in renal biopsy. Doppler ultrasound of renal vessels is a useful way of detecting blood flow in transplanted kidneys and may soon become available for the analysis of blood flow in normal and diseased kidneys.

CT scan

This may be used to define retroperitoneal masses, secondary deposits and, rarely, intra-renal masses.

2.6 Procedures using isotopic techniques

Renography

Depending on which isotope is used, different types of renogram may be obtained.

1 Technetium-labelled di-ethylenetriamine penta-acetic acid (DTPA) for normal γ camera renogram.

2 Technetium-labelled dimercaptosuccinic acid (DMSA) for better parenchymal resolution.

3 Radio-iodine hippuran for renography in patients with renal failure.

Renography can define the site and size of the kidneys, assess function, and assist with the diagnosis of obstruction or renal artery stenosis. It is possible also to determine residual bladder capacity and vesico-ureteric reflux.

Other tests undertaken by the nuclear medicine department are shown in Table 2.2.

Table 2.2 Tests undertaken by the nuclear medicine department.

Measurement	Isotope	Comments
Plasma volume	^{125}I Human serum albumin	Can be
Extracellular fluid	^{77}Br	mixed and
Total body sodium	^{24}Na	individual
Total body potassium	^{43}K	spaces computed

2.7 Renal biopsy

Renal biopsy has become an integral part of the assessment of renal pathology.

Contraindications

Most physicians would be hesitant to biopsy those patients with:

- a single kidney
- a bleeding diathesis

- small kidneys, advanced diabetic glomerulosclerosis or untreated malignant hypertension
- active urinary infection or suspected neoplasm

Preparation
1 Full blood count (FBC), platelets, prothrombin time, kaolin cephalin clotting time (KCCT), bleeding time, hepatitis B antigen. Save serum for group and cross-match.
2 Correction of a prolonged prothrombin time (INR> 1.3) or a prolonged bleeding time (> 10 minutes) may be undertaken with fresh frozen plasma or DDAVP (0.3 μg/kg) respectively.

Method
The biopsy may be undertaken 'blind' or in association with either X-ray screening or ultrasound. The patient is positioned prone on a firm pillow and local anaesthetic is infiltrated down to the kidney capsule. This gives some idea of the depth involved. Biopsy is undertaken on the lateral body of the left (easier) kidney (Chapter 1), using either a Franklin Silvermann or Tru-cut needle. Recently a biopsy gun has been introduced into which a Tru-cut needle can be inserted giving a less traumatic section. Sufficient material should be obtained for light, immune and electron microscopy study.

Post-biopsy management
The pulse and blood pressure should be monitored for 24 hours following biopsy. The patient should be supine and encouraged to drink at least 1 litre of water. Patients often experience some pain and a small amount of haematuria is to be expected.

2.8 Bladder function tests

Assessment of bladder function is becoming an important part of the investigation of urinary symptoms, such as unexplained frequency or incontinence or where bladder neck obstruction is suspected. Assessment is based on a thorough clinical examination together with the use of various techniques of increasing sophistication:

- monitoring of the flow of urine, where a time-rate and volume curve may be obtained
- urethral and bladder pressure profile
- video-cystourethrography

In video-cystourethrography, a combined filling volume, intravesical pressure, detrusor pressure, flow rate, rectal pressure and voiding volume, may be obtained. Data are recorded on videotape for later examination. Residual urine volume (normally less than 50 ml) and reflux may be detected.

2.9 Urinalysis

This includes:
- the direct examination of urine using 'stick' tests
- direct microscopy to examine for cells, casts and crystals

Urine should be collected by the *mid-stream technique* whatever examination is to be used. Suprapubic aspiration of the bladder is useful in children and for accurate assessment of possible infection at whatever age.

Stick tests

There are a number of commercially available chemically impregnated paper strips which test for different constituents in urine. Some of the problems with stick tests are set out in Table 2.3.

Other tests for protein
1 25% salicyl sulphonic acid is added drop by drop to urine containing a protein, it results in a precipitate. If the urine is initially cloudy, acetic acid should be added first. This test is sensitive to a level of 300 mg/dl.
2 Boiling test for protein is now rarely used.
3 There must be 24-hour collection for accurate quantitation.

Microscopy of urine

The examination of fresh, unspun urine for red and white blood cells and centrifuged urine for casts and crystals is an

Table 2.3 Problems with stick tests in urinalysis

Test	Comments	False-positive	False-negative
Protein	Sensitive to 20 mg/dl (i.e. within normal range)	Alkaline buffers, quaternary ammonium compounds	Less sensitive for globulin and Bence–Jones protein
Blood	Sensitivity reduced in concentrated urine	Hypochlorite, urinary infection (rare), myoglobinuria	Cannot distinguish haemaglobinuria from haematuria
pH	Avoid contamination from protein area of stick		
Glucose	Specific for glucose		Rarely, large amount of ketones
Ketones	Positive with aceto-acetic acid and acetone	Presence of bromosulphthalein, phenylketones or L-Dopa metabolites	Does not react with β-hydroxybutyric acid
Bilirubin	Specific in concentration of $> 3.4–6.8$ μmol	Chlorpromazine, pyridium	
Urobilinogen	Not reliable for porphobilinogen	Any drug with diazo dye	
Nitrate (for bacteria)	Gram-negative organism in concentration of $> 10^5$/ml	Heavy contamination	Gram-positive organisms

important part of the assessment of patients with a variety of renal diseases. The examination can be done in out-patients or in a renal laboratory with a binocular microscope fitted with phase contrast and a counting chamber.

Red and white blood cells

These are present in normal unspun mid-stream urine in a concentration of less than $10/cm^3$. The finding of excess red and white cells should be verified and the patient investigated if confirmed.

The origin of red cells may be differentiated by morphology and size. The appearances of glomular and non-glomular red cells is given in Figure 2.4.

Some likely causes of symptomless excess white cells (pyuria) and haematuria are given in Table 2.4.

Casts

These are best examined in centrifuged samples. Improved resolution may be obtained by using stains, e.g. Steinheimers.

Hyaline casts occur in normal individuals, with febrile illnesses, after exercise and are of limited diagnostic value.

Granular casts are always pathological and indicate glomerular damage. They are seen in glomerulonephritis, diabetic glomerulo-sclerosis, and amyloidosis.

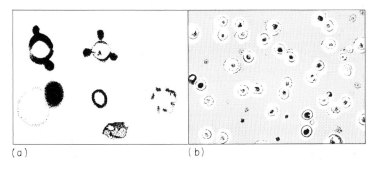

(a)   (b)

Fig. 2.4 Common variety of (a) glomular; and (b) non-glomular red cells.

Table 2.4 Causes of symptomless excess white cells and haematuria.

Pyuria	Haematuria
Contamination	Contamination
Urinary tract infections	Bladder neoplasms
Calculi	Renal and pelvic neoplasms
Neoplasms	Glomerulonephritis
Tuberculosis	Calculi
Analgesic nephropathy	Bleeding diathesis
Glomerulonephritis	Polycystic kidney
	Schistosomiasis

Red cell casts indicate glomerular damage and are typically seen with acute glomerulonephritis.

In summary, examination of urine for casts is a useful method of screening for renal disease, especially glomerulonephritis. In nearly every instance haematuria and heavy proteinuria are found as well.

Crystals
The presence of crystals is of limited diagnostic importance. Urine should be fresh and warm if *oxalate* crystals are to be detected (Fig. 2.5), but cool if hexagonal *cystine* crystals are to be found (Fig. 2.6).

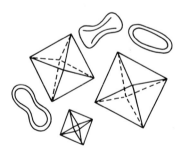

Fig. 2.5 Oxalate crystals.

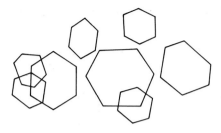

Fig. 2.6 Cystine crystals.

Urinary bacteriology

Direct microscopy of urine collected by a mid-stream technique cannot be used to assess the presence of bacteria since it is impossible to differentiate bacteriuria (the presence of viable organisms in the bladder urine) from urethral and vestibular contamination. In contrast, the presence of organisms in urine obtained by suprapubic aspiration indicates bacteriuria.

Culture of urine

Urine may be cultured by a variety of techniques including a standard 'loop', filter paper method, or by using dip inoculum methods. The ability to culture urine in a renal laboratory, can prove extremely useful in the management of patients with suspected urinary infection.

3: The kidney and electrolyte disorders

3.1 Control of water excretion

Water excretion is governed by the level of circulating anti-diuretic hormone (ADH, vasopressin), an octapeptide secreted by the hypothalamus. The level of circulating ADH is regulated by osmolar and non-osmolar forces. Increasing plasma osmolality stimulates ADH release and decreasing plasma osmolality inhibits ADH release. Non-osmolar forces act through the autonomic nervous system and include stress (which inhibits ADH release), adrenal insufficiency, and cardiac failure (both of which stimulate ADH release). ADH enhances water reabsorption at the collecting duct and any functional or structural abnormality of the collecting duct will alter renal concentrating (or diluting) capacity.

3.2 Control of sodium excretion

The normal kidney can adjust the excretion of sodium to as little as 1–2 mmol per day with salt restriction, or several hundred mmol following a salt load. In contrast to the mechanisms of water excretion, sodium excretion is poorly understood. The afferent arc includes changes in extracellular fluid (ECF) volume, viscosity, cardiac output, venous capacitance acting on pressure-sensitive receptors in the great veins, atria, and carotid bodies. Efferent signals are relayed to the kidney via changes in the GFR, certain intra-renal physical factors, aldosterone and other hormones such as prostaglandins, and natriuretic hormones including atrial natriuretic peptide (ANP).

3.3 Disorders of water and salt regulation

Both renal and extra-renal disorders produce abnormalities in the volume and concentration of body water and salt. Abnormalities often occur together but may occur independently. It is important to realise that serum sodium is not proportional to body sodium but is influenced by water regulation.

Polyuria

Patients with polyuria present an interesting problem to the nephrologist. The main causes include:
- polyuria due to osmotic diuresis, e.g. diabetes mellitus
- diabetes insipidus
- compulsive water drinking
- loss of renal concentrating ability:
    (a) structural: e.g. obstruction, papillary necrosis, medullary cystic disease, chronic renal failure
    (b) functional: nephrogenic diabetes insipidus, drugs (e.g. demethylchlortetracycline), hypercalcaemia and hypo-kalaemia

The distinction between diabetes insipidus, compulsive water drinking and nephrogenic diabetes insipidus is easily established by a combination of water deprivation and vasopressin administration. Patients with compulsive water drinking should concentrate their urine normally in response to both dehydration and vasopressin, those with diabetes insipidus to vasopressin alone and those with nephrogenic diabetes insipidus to neither test. In practice, considerable overlap exists between the tests but as a rough guide the maximum urine concentrations to be expected are shown in Table 3.1. *It is important to monitor the patient carefully (weigh 2-hourly) and stop water deprivation if more than 5% of body weight is*

Table 3.1 Maximum urine concentration mmol/kg water.

Condition	Water deprivation	Vasopressin test	Percentage change
Normal	1200	1000	−9
Diabetes insipidus	No change	450	+180
Compulsive water drinking	750	780	+5
Nephrogenic diabetes insipidus	No change	No change	

lost. Details of the tests themselves are given on p. 205.

Note that the *percentage change* is more important than the absolute values. Thus, an increase in urine osmolality of greater than 10% after vasopressin, compared to after water deprivation, is more likely due to diabetes insipidus, partial or complete. A reliable radioimmune assay of vasopressin will help to differentiate these cases further, aided by saline infusion and measurement of urine flow rate (Zerbe and Robinson (1981) *New England Journal of Medicine* **305**, 1539).

Hypernatraemia
(plasma sodium concentration > 145 mmol/l)
In states of both hyponatraemia and hypernatraemia it is important to assess
- the state of hydration
- the urinary sodium loss
- any drugs (particularly i.v. infusions) the patient is receiving
- co-existing hepatic, cardiac or renal disease

The causes and treatment of various hypernatraemia states are given in Table 3.2.

Severe hypernatraemia is rare and usually results from iatrogenic manipulations, e.g. administration of 2 N saline or attempted dehydration of patients with diabetes insipidus. Hypernatraemia leads to cellular dehydration, neurological sequelae (restlessness, ataxia, fits, coma) cerebellar haemorrhage, hypertension and death.

Hyponatraemia
(plasma sodium concentration < 130 mmol/l)
In contrast to hypernatraemia, hyponatraemia occurs frequently in any hospital. The principle causes and management are set out in Table 3.2.

Hyponatraemia also has profound neuropsychiatric sequelae associated with cerebral oedema. Symptoms include anorexia, vomiting, restlessness, disturbed conciousness, increased reflexes, confusion, fits and grades of coma. These features are more likely to develop in elderly subjects and with acute, rather than chronic, changes.

It is vital to correct hyponatraemia *slowly* particularly in older female patients with long-standing hyponatraemia. Rapid correction may lead to pontine myelinolysis. During the initial 48 hours normo and hypernatraemia must be avoided and the plasma sodium rasied by less than 25 mmol/l. Frequent (2−4 hourly) measurements of plasma sodium are mandatory.

For both hyponatraemia and hypernatraemia the amount of water to be lost or gained can be calculated from the following equation:

$$\text{Desired water loss (or gain)} = \frac{\text{Actual plasma sodium}}{\text{Desired plasma sodium}}$$
$$\times \text{(TBW} = 60\% \text{ of body weight)}$$

NB This assumes the patient is euvolaemic.

Side-effects of diuretics

1 Volume depletion with hyponatraemia, occurring in elderly patients with co-existent cardiac or liver disease. There is impairment of renal diluting capacity (reduced free-water clearance) but urinary sodium concentration remains elevated. *Treatment* is by reducing water intake, and, if hyponatraemia is profound (plasma sodium concentration less than 120 mmol/l) or neuropsychiatric complications occur, by infusing 2 N saline and the cautious administration of frusemide in an attempt to increase free-water clearance. *Prevention* lies in careful monitoring of diuretic therapy with regular checks of blood pressure, weight and electrolytes especially if there is intermittent illness, e.g. gastroenteritis. NB hyponatraemia must be corrected slowly (see above).

2 Other complications include hypokalaemia, a metabolic acidosis, carbohydrate intolerance, hyperuricaemia and, rarely, hypercalcaemia.

3 Some women take diuretics for alleged ankle oedema. It has been shown that, in these women, oedema may worsen with continued diuretic abuse. Cessation of the diuretic leads, after

Table 3.2 Causes and treatment of hypernatraemic and hyponatraemic states.

Cause	Total body sodium	Urinary sodium concentration (mmol/l)	Treatment
Hypernatraemia			
Sodium and water deprivation			
Renal: osmotic diuresis	Low	> 20 ⎱	Hypotonic saline
Extra-renal, e.g. sweating	Low	< 10 ⎰	
Water deprivation			
Renal or central diabetes insipidus*	Normal	Variable ⎱	Water replacement
Extra-renal, e.g. sweating (rare)	Normal	Variable ⎰	
Absolute gain in sodium			
Hypertonic saline* ⎱	Increased	> 20	Diuretics and water
Hyperaldosteronism ⎰			
Hyponatraemia			
More salt than water loss			
Renal			
Diuretic excess* ⎱	Low	> 20	Give isotonic saline
Addison's disease			
Renal tubular acidosis			
Osmotic diuresis ⎰			

Cause			Treatment
Extra-renal Vomiting Diarrhoea	Low	< 10	Give isotonic saline
Water retention Addison's disease Hypothyroidism Inappropriate ADH secretion* (SIADH) HIV infection Drugs, e.g. chlorpropamide Misuse of dextrose saline*	Increased	> 20	Treat underlying disease Stop drugs Restrict water, demethylchlortetracycline 300 mg t.d.s. (for SIADH)
Less salt than water retention Nephrotic syndrome Cirrhosis Cardiac failure*	Increased (oedema)	< 10	Restrict water
Acute and chronic renal failure	Increased	> 20	Restrict water

* Common causes
(Note pseudohyponatraemia in the plasma with serum lipids.)

a few days of further salt and water retention, to a satisfactory naturesis and diuresis.

4 Diuretic abuse may present a bizarre clinical picture resembling Barrter's syndrome. There is profound hypokalaemia, increased urinary sodium and potassium loss with a normal blood pressure. However, aldosterone is raised in Barrter's syndrome, (secondary to increased renin) but reduced in diuretic abuse (secondary to reduced plasma potassium) see p. 189.

5 Certain diuretics have specific side-effects: hyperkalaemia with potassium-sparing drugs (spironolactone, amiloride, and triamterene), especially in patients with renal failure; interstitial nephritis (rare) with thiazide diuretics and frusemide; rashes and granulocytopenia with thiazide diuretics; and deafness with large doses of ethacrynic acid (rare) and frusemide (very rare).

Syndrome of inappropriate secretion of ADH (SIADH)

This presents with hyponatraemia, low plasma osmolality and inapproriately high urinary osmolality. There are a number of causes, including:
- malignancies, (lung, pancreas)
- lung disorders, e.g. pneumonia
- central nervous system (CNS) disorders, e.g. encephalitis, cerebrovascular accidents, brain abscess, trauma

Clinical features
These are those of hyponatraemia and treatment is aimed at affecting the underlying conditions, restricting water and giving demethylchlortetracycline (300 mg t.d.s.).

3.4 Control of potassium excretion

In contrast to sodium, the kidney has limited power of potassium conservation. Potassium levels are determined by intake, catabolism (e.g. muscle breakdown) aldosterone levels, sodium intake and intracellular H^+ ion concentration.

3.5 Disorders of potassium excretion

Hyperkalaemia

(plasma potassium concentration > 5.5 mmol/l)
This is the most dangerous of all electrolyte disturbances in patients with renal failure. The insidious onset, lack of clinical manifestation and disastrous consequences, demand prompt action and continuous observation.

Causes and associated conditions
- acute and chronic renal failure
- potassium supplements, diet, drugs
- acidosis
- potassium-sparing diuretics (spironolactone, amiloride, triamterene)
- Addison's disease
- low renin hypoaldosteronism (see 68)
- false hyperkalaemia: tourniquets, haemolysis, increased white cell or platelet count

Symptoms and signs
Weakness, abdominal pain, vomiting, arrhythmia, cardiac arrest.

ECG changes
- peaked T waves in precordial leads
- reduced R wave amplitude, widening QRS
- increased PR interval
- QRS blends with T waves
- ventricular fibrillation or asystole

Treatment
Plasma potassium concentration 5.5–6.0 mmol/l
- stop potassium supplements
- if patient not fluid-overloaded, administer resonium A 15–30 g b.d.–t.d.s. orally or rectally
- if patient fluid-overloaded, administer calcium resin 15–30 g b.d.–t.d.s. orally or rectally

Plasma potassium concentration 6.0−7.0 mmol/l
- stop potassium supplements
- administer resonium A or calcium resins, as above.
- i.v. β agonist (e.g. salbutamol 10 mg over 6 hours)
- sodium bicarbonate, e.g. 500 ml 1.2%, or 250 ml 2.4%, i.v. in 4 hours; use with care as this may produce hypocalcaemia
- 70% Sorbitol 50−100 ml orally (particularly useful if patient fluid-overloaded).

Plasma potassium concentration > 7.0 mmol/l
- stop potassium supplements
- administer resonium A or calcium resin, as above
- sodium bicarbonate, as above
- 70% Sorbitol 100 ml orally
- give calcium supplements, e.g. 20 ml 10% calcium gluconate i.v.
- 50% glucose 100 ml and insulin 20 u i.v. in 30 min
- dialyse

Dialysis, if available, should take preference over other forms of treatment.

Hypokalaemia
(plasma potassium concentration < 3.5 mmol/l)
This is a rare accompaniment of renal disease. Important causes of hypokalaemia include the following.
1 Gastro-intestinal losses: vomiting, diarrhoea, laxatives.
2 Renal causes: diuretics, renal tubular acidosis, overzealous dialysis with low dialysate potassium.
3 Endocrine (via renal loss): aldosteronism, Barrter's syndrome, Cushing's disease and steroid treatment, adrenocorticotrophic hormone (ACTH) producing tumours, liqorice.
4 Rare causes: familial periodic paralysis, inadequate diet, β_2 agonists (e.g. salbutamol).

Effects
These include skeletal muscle weakness, ileus, arrhythmias and orthostatic hypotension. A urinary potassium concentration

above 20 mmol/l is suggestive of renal potassium loss or an acute gastro-intestinal loss. A urinary potassium concentration of less than 20 mmol/l suggests a chronic gastro-intestinal loss. The notion that hypokalaemia by itself results in an increased renal loss of potassium has not been upheld, especially when the hypokalaemia is long-standing. Hypokalaemia increases urinary ammonium excretion and also raises urine pH. The association between hypertension and hypokalaemia is discussed on p. 184.

Treatment
- treat underlying causes
- replace potassium chloride orally
- if profound (plasma potassium concentration < 2.0 mmol/l), and associated with vomiting, potassium chloride may be given i.v. *but never more than 10 mmol per hour.* If larger doses are required cardiac monitoring is essential.

3.6 The kidney and acid-base balance

The kidney provides an important role in the regulation of acid-base balance, conserving bicarbonate in respiratory acidosis, excreting H^+ ions in non-renal metabolic acidosis and bicarbonate in metabolic alkalosis. In all these compensatory mechanisms renal function is otherwise intact. Metabolic acidosis may be conveniently divided into two groups according to the anion gap $[Na - (Cl + HCO_3)]$ (Table 3.3).

Table 3.3 Metabolic acidosis.

Normal gap (8–12)	Increased gap
Renal tubular acidosis	Lactic acidosis
Tubulo interstitial disease	Diabetes mellitus
Ammonium chloride administration	Renal failure
Diarrhoea	
Ureterosigmoidostomy	

Metabolic acidosis may be associated with a paradoxical alkaline urine, a group of conditions known as renal tubular acidosis (RTA). These result from either a failure to excrete H^+ ions (type 1, distal RTA) or proximal tubular bicarbonate wastage (type 2, proximal RTA). Both result in a hyperchloraemic acidosis with a high urinary pH. A summary of the 2 main types of renal tubular acidosis is given in Table 3.4. A useful nomogram for the assessment of acid-base status in a particular patient is given in Figure 3.1.

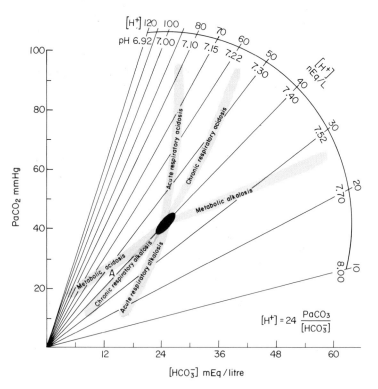

Fig. 3.1 Nomogram of acid-base balance (after Henderson). This nomogram allows for a rapid assessment of acid-base status. In particular it allows: (a) correct assessment of the relation between pH, P_{CO_2} and bicarbonate; and (b) pure changes follow the hatched areas, whereas mixed changes lie between hatched areas, e.g. **A** is mixed metabolic acidosis and respiratory alkalosis. (Courtesy Professor A Guz).

Table 3.4 Renal tubular acidosis.

	Type 1 (distal tubular acidosis)	Type 2 (proximal tubular acidosis)
Mechanism	Failure to produce H$^+$ ion gradiant in distal tubule	Bicarbonate wastage from proximal tubule
Causes	Primary: 　sporadic or inherited associated with 　autoimmune disorder, 　Sjögren's, 　hypergammaglobulinaemia Medullary sponge kidney Nephrocalcinosis	Hyperparathyroidism Proximal tubule poisoning Heavy metals, e.g. cadmium Primary Amyloidosis Myeloma
Ammonium chloride test	Urine pH always >5.4	Normal response (pH <5.4)
X-ray appearance	Related to underlying disease, nephrocalcinosis Osteomalacia, hypokalaemia	Related to underlying disease, no nephrocalcinosis Other proximal tubule wastage, e.g. glucose, phosphate, amino acids.
Treatment	Sodium bicarbonate or potassium citrate 60–200 mmol per day	Underlying disorder, large doses of bicarbonate will not correct acidosis

3.7 Hypercalcaemia and hypocalcaemia

Disorders of calcium and phosphate metabolism in chronic renal disease are discussed in Chapter 5. It is convenient to mention hypercalcaemia and hypocalcaemia among electrolyte disturbances. In any disorder of serum calcium, it is important to check the serum albumin (see Appendix 5) for correction factor) and, if possible, to measure the ionized calcium level.

Hypercalcaemia

(plasma calcium concentration > 2.6 mmol/l)
Hypercalcaemia can result from a number of causes (Table 3.5).

Table 3.5 Causes of hypercalcaemia.

Causes	Associated features
Hyperparathyroidism	Low plasma phosphate; ↑ urinary phosphate; metabolic acidosis; ↑ PTH
Sarcoidosis	↑ Ca^{2+} absorption (?) secondary to ↑ 1−25 $(OH)_2$ vitamin D_3; ↓ PTH
Vitamin D intoxication	More likely and more prolonged with ergocalciferol, or calciferol
Neoplastic diseases	PTH ↑ or normal, prostaglandin mediated (?)
Milk-alkali syndrome	↑ Plasma phosphate, metastatic calcification
Hyperthyroidism	↑ Bone turnover
Immobilization	Especially in children and adolescents

↑ : Increased;   ↓ : Decreased;   PTH: parathyroid hormone.

Effects
Hypercalcaemia is often symptomless but may result in vomiting, pruritus, red eyes, renal failure and ECG changes (shortened QRT interval prolonged P−R interval).

Treatment
- treatment of the underlying condition
- rehydration with saline (helps saline depletion due to vomiting and improves renal function)
- induced calcium diuresis by saline and frusemide, e.g. 1 litre saline 4 hourly +20 mg frusemide i.v. The weight of the patient must be kept constant and plasma potassium measured frequently
- disodium etidronate (7.5 mg i.v. daily for 3 days, followed by 20 mg per kg orally for 30 days if necessary)
- indomethacin (25−50 mg t.d.s.) may be useful for hypercalcaemia associated with malignancies
- calcium absorption may be blunted with cellulose phosphate or sodium phytate
- steroids (prednisolone 60 mg daily in divided doses) may be given for vitamin D intoxication, sarcoidosis and malignancy
- calcitonin — slow and not very effective
- haemo or peritoneal dialysis with calcium-free solution

NB i.v. phosphate produces widespread metastatic calcification and should not be given.

Hypocalcaemia

(plasma calcium concentration < 2.2 mmol/l)
Causes of hypocalcaemia include:
- vitamin D deficiency: dietary, malabsorption, liver enzyme induction, nephrotic syndrome
- renal disease: acute or chronic renal failure
- other causes: hypoparathyroidism (particularly post-parathyroidectomy), pseudohypoparathyroidism, calcitonin-producing tumours

Clinical features
Oral paraesthasiae, tetany, proximal myopathy (if associated with osteomalacia), brisk jerks, positive Chvostek's and Trousseau's signs, are all features. Dangerous hypocalcaemia may occasionally be associated with ECG changes (prolonged QT interval) or even cardiac arrest.

Treatment
- treat the underlying disease
- give calcium supplements, e.g. calcium lactate i.v., oral calcium carbonate (e.g. Titralac or Calcichew)
- give vitamin D, e.g. $1-25(OH)_2D_3$ (calcitriol) in small doses, (starting at 0.25 μg b.d.) and monitoring serum calcium and phosphate

3.8 Hypermagnesaemia and hypomagnesaemia

(plasma magnesium concentration >1.0 or <0.7 mmol/l respectively)

Hypermagnesaemia

This is a rare accompaniment of renal failure occurring when patients with renal failure are given magnesium salts (usually as antacids). It may rarely be associated with adrenal insufficiency. Clinical features include weakness, even progressing to quadriplegia and respiratory depression.

Treatment
- for severe hypermagnesaemia give calcium salts, e.g. 5–10 mEq of Ca lactate i.v.
- stop magnesium supplements
- dialyse with magnesium-free dialysate

Table 3.6 Causes of hypomagnesaemia.

Cause	Effect
Malabsorption Protein calorie malnutrition Alcoholism	Low urinary magnesium
Diabetes ketoacidosis Diuretics Hyperaldosteronism	High urinary magnesium
Vitamin D treatment Primary hyperparathyroidism	Miscellaneous

Hypomagnesaemia

This is only rarely associated with renal disease. There are numerous causes including those given in Table 3.6.

Clinical features
Weakness, fasciculation, tremor, tetany, positive Chvostek's or Trousseau's sign, delirium, psychoses.

Treatment
Replace magnesium with magnesium salts, e.g. magnesium sulphate 5 g in 10 ml i.v. (20.4 mmol) or orally.

4: Acute renal failure (ARF)

4.1 Introduction

Definitions of acute renal failure vary, but encompass a rapidly rising blood urea and plasma creatinine concentration and, usually, a falling urinary output. *Oliguria* is a urine output of less than 400 ml per 24 hours. *Anuria* no urine at all. Some patients with ARF have high (up to 21 per day) urine outputs (polyuric acute renal failure).

Acute tubular necrosis

This is a histological entity which correlates poorly with renal function.

Clinical assessment

When a patient is first seen with apparent acute renal failure two questions need to be asked.
1 Is the patient suffering from acute renal failure?
2 Does the patient need urgent medical attention?
As far as question 1 is concerned it is important to exclude dehydration ('pre-renal' failure) and obstruction ('post-renal' failure). Question 2 demands quick clinical decisions, especially if the patient has severe volume overload or hyperkalaemia. The important decisions in the management of patients with ARF are shown in Fig. 4.1.

4.2 Differentiation between ARF and dehydration

Although this may appear superficially easy, in practice it can be extraordinarily difficult. Classical diagnostic features, together with some biochemical abnormalities, are given in Table 4.1.

Some authorities believe that there are patients with 'pre-renal' failure and that the administration of frusemide

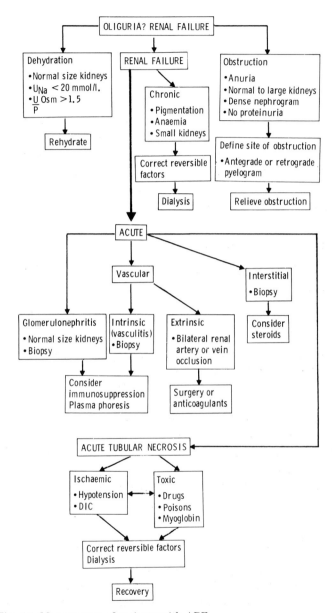

Fig. 4.1 Management of patients with ARF.

Table 4.1 Diagnostic features of ARF and dehydration.

Feature	Acute renal failure	Dehydration
Oedema	Variable	Absent
JVP/CVP	Low, normal or raised	Low or normal (unless concurrent heart failure)
Blood pressure	Variable	Low, especially on standing
Urine protein	Positive or negative (with obstruction)	Negative
U/P osmolality	< 1.1	> 1.5
Urine sodium concentration mmol/l	> 40	< 20
Urine urea concentration mmol/l	< 150	> 150
Fractional excretion of sodium	> 1%	< 1%

$$\text{Fractional excretion of sodium} = \frac{\text{Urinary sodium} \times \text{plasma creatinine} \times 100}{\text{Plasma sodium} \times \text{urinary creatinine}}$$

(80–120 mg i.v.) or mannitol (100 ml of 20%) may prevent the development of overt tubular necrosis. The evidence for this is meagre and frusemide may worsen dehydration. However, there is some evidence that frusemide given to patients with acute renal failure produces a small diuresis which, although not reducing the need for dialysis, may enable extra fluid to be given.

4.3 Investigation of established ARF

Once it has been established that the patient is suffering from ARF an attempt should be made to define the cause, and in particular to exclude obstruction. This involves a careful history and physical examination, noting any previous urinary tract problems, renal calculi, drug history, recent surgery, blood transfusion, trauma, the presence of pallor, oedema, jaundice, blood pressure, cardiomegally, signs of salt and water overload, or hepatosplenomegaly, rectal and vaginal examination, peripheral pulses.

Whatever the suspected cause of ARF, the following investigations should be undertaken.

1 Blood tests for full blood count, film, platelet count, fibrin degradation products, urea, electrolytes, creatinine, creatinine kinase, calcium, phosphorus, liver function tests, glucose, osmolality, hepatitis B antigen, antistreptolysin O (ASO) titre, antinuclear factor (ANF), blood culture.

2 Urine tests for microscopy, culture and sensitivity, protein, urea, sodium, creatinine, osmolality, haemoglobin and myoglobin.

3 Assessment of renal size by ultrasound or plain X-ray (tomography of renal areas).

4 Assessment of renal function by isotope renography.

5 Obstruction must be ruled out by urography, ultrasound, antegrade pyelogram (preferably), retrograde pyelogram (rarely).

6 Renal biopsy should be considered (for preparation see Chapter 2). This is used to exclude intrinsic renal disease including *acute interstitial nephritis*. This differentiation is important, since acute interstitial nephritis may respond to

prednisolone and rapidly progressive glomerulonephritis (including Goodpasture's syndrome, see p. 88), and acute vasculitis with acute renal failure may respond to immunosuppressives or plasmaphoresis. Acute interstitial nephritis is associated with fever, eosinophilia, rash, eosinophiluria and is most likely caused by one of the drugs shown in Table 4.2.

Table 4.2 Drugs causing interstitial nephritis.

Commonly	Rarely
Methicillin	Frusemide
Ampicillin	Penicillin
Rifampicin	Flucloxacillin
Phenindione	Phenylbutazone
Sulphonamides	Sulphinpyrazone

Renal size and ARF

Different kidney sizes (established with urography or ultrasound) indicate the following:
• normal: acute tubular necrosis, obstruction, myeloma, diabetes, amyloidosis, polyarteritis
• bilateral small kidneys: chronic renal failure
• large kidneys: amyloidosis, renal vein thrombosis, bilateral hydronephrosis, polycystic kidneys, acute glomerulonephritis, acute interstitial nephritis
• unequal size (>1.5 cm difference): previous obstruction, reflux nephropathy, papillary necrosis (rare), renal vascular disease (rare)

An increasing denseness in nephrogram indicates obstruction.

Renography

This may help to show renal size, vascularity, (major renal artery occlusion) and outflow tract obstruction.

4.4 Causes of established ARF

A comprehensive list of likely causes is of limited value. However, general categories with a few examples are shown here.

Impaired vascular supply
This may be due to aortic occlusion, bilateral renal artery occlusion, or bilateral renal vein thrombosis. These conditions are rare but major arterial occlusions occur in patients with severe atheroma, dissection of the aorta, or mitral valve disease (arterial emboli). Diagnosis of aortic occlusion is made by aortography. Renal vein thrombosis may complicate renal amyloid, membranous glomerulonephritis or, rarely, other intrinsic renal disease.

Toxic renal damage ('acute tubular necrosis')
Toxic renal damage can be caused by hypotension (blood loss, heart disease), drugs (e.g. aminoglycosides, amphoteracin), poisons (e.g. mercuric chloride, carbon tetrachloride), intravascular coagulation (e.g. septicaemia, post-partum acute renal failure), haemolysis (e.g. transfusion reactions, drugs and G6PD deficiency), myoglobinuria (traumatic and non-traumatic).

This group comprises the bulk of patients seen with ARF. In any one patient there is often more than one cause, e.g. a sick post-operative patient may be suffering from hypotension, sepsis, liver failure, effects of nephrotoxic drugs, poor cardiac output and intravascular coagulation.

Intrinsic renal disease
This includes acute glomerulonephritis, rapidly progressive glomerulonephritis, acute interstitial nephritis, acute pyelonephritis (very rare) and acute vasculitis. Pointers to intrinsic renal disease include oedema, hypoproteinaemia, haematuria, proteinuria, granular and red cell casts and normal size kidneys. Vasculitic lesions of the skin may be amenable to biopsy.

Obstruction
Bilateral renal calculi (maybe non-opaque), bilateral papillary necrosis with impacted calcified papillae, retroperitoneal

fibrosis, carcinoma of the bladder, prostate, cervix or large bowel, may cause obstruction. ARF can be induced by obstructions anywhere in the urinary tract, from the urethra to the renal pelvis. The presence of a large bladder, pelvic or rectal masses, prostatic hypertrophy or malignancy, suggest lower urinary tract obstruction. Bilateral upper urinary tract obstruction is rare. Anuria or lack of proteinuria are pointers towards upper urinary tract obstruction.

Hepato-renal syndrome
This is characterized by oliguria, renal failure, *low* urinary sodium concentration (less than 10 mmol/l), increased urine osmolality without proteinuria, occurring in patients with hepatic failure usually due to advanced cirrhosis. Sodium and water conservation is intact and distinguishes the hepato-renal syndrome from acute renal failure in patients with liver disease when urinary sodium would exceed 20 mmol/l. The cause is unknown. Treatment is difficult but cautious volume expansion, and recirculation of ascites either by reinfusion or with a peritoneal jugular venous shunt, has been tried with some success. Various drugs (phenoxybenzamine, dopamine, mannitol and vasodilators) have given disappointing results.

4.5 Management

This will depend on the severity of the renal failure and co-existing problems. A few (especially polyuric) patients will require conservative management only, providing that there is no fluid overload, hyperkalaemia or other electrolyte imbalance, e.g. hyponatraemia (water overload).

Conservative management

- withdrawal of nephrotoxic agents
- correction of fluid balance — usually achieved by keeping the optimum weight constant with 500 ml of fluid plus the equivalent of the previous day's output of urine and gastro-intestinal losses (e.g. diarrhoea and vomit losses)
- monitoring of electrolyte balance with daily electrolytes,

urea and creatinine; avoidance of high sodium or potassium intake including drugs
- regular (twice daily) weight and blood pressure
- adequate nutrition with a minimum of 2000 kcal per day plus sufficient minerals and vitamins
- 60 g protein diet until urea starts to fall, then normal protein intake
- prophylactic antacid, e.g. Aludrox 20 ml t.d.s. to prevent acute gastric erosion from bleeding
- prompt treatment of any infections
- removal of urinary catheter as soon as possible
- dopamine 2–3 micrograms $kg^{-1}min^{-1}$ improves renal blood flow

When to dialyse?

There are no hard and fast rules. In general, the aim is to keep the patient as fit as possible and allow adequate nutrition. Short daily dialysis may be required for a sick hypercatabolic patient, less frequent dialysis for patients with lower levels of urea and creatinine. In general, the aim is to keep the urea below 30 mmol/l and creatinine below 500 µmol/l.

4.6 Types of dialysis

Haemo and peritoneal dialysis for patients with acute renal failure are gradually being superseded by either continuous arteriovenous (CAVH) or venovenous (CVVH) haemofiltration or more recently by continuous arteriovenous or venovenous haemodialysis (CAVHD or CVVHD). The advantage of these techniques lies in their simplicity requiring no special instrumental monitoring, better cardiovascular stability and non-dependence on renal unit staffing.

Continuous haemofiltration is undertaken using either arteriovenous access (shunts or femoral catheters) or venovenous access (subclavian or internal jugular or femoral vein catheters). AV access is preferable since no circulating pumps are required. Highly porous dialysers are used (e.g. Gambro filters) but high volumes of fluid (up to 1 litre per hour) have to be ultrafiltered to maintain urea and creatinine levels below 30 mmol/l and 500 µmol/l respectively.

Continuous arteriovenous haemodialysis (CAVHD) is undertaken using dialysers with highly porous membranes (e.g. Hospal AN60 or Fresenius F60) with low ultrafiltration rates (approximately 2 litres per 24 hours and low (1–2 litres per hour) dialysis flow rates (Fig. 4.2). Initially 2 litres per hour dialysis flows are used but once the urea is brought down to 25 mmol/l, 1 litre dialytic flows are usually sufficient. The dialyser will need changing every 48–72 hours and at 1 litre per hour dialysate flow rate, the dialysate urea equals the blood urea.

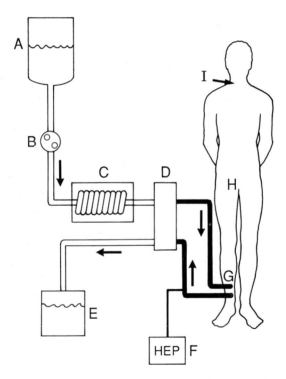

Fig. 4.2 Continuous arterio- or veno-venous haemodialysis. Peritoneal dialysis fluid is run in from A, through pump B and warming coil C, to dialyser D and collected in E. Blood access is obtained either by a shunt G, femoral lines H or neck line I. Heparin is infused at F.

Conventional haemodialysis may still be required in certain highly catabolic patients and is best undertaken by trained renal unit nurses. *Peritoneal dialysis* is occasionally useful in patients with bleeding problems or with pancreatitis but is not as effective as dialysis and may result in peritonitis, protein loss and secondary chest infection.

4.7 Technique of acute peritoneal dialysis

Preparation

The bladder should be emptied, with a catheter if necessary. Some physicians prefer to run 1 litre of dialysis fluid into the abdomen at this stage through a small needle.

Procedure

The peritoneal catheter should be inserted through a small stab incision by an aseptic technique, in the lower abdomen, either in the midline or in the flank if there is an old midline scar. Insertion is easier if the patient's head is elevated slightly to stretch the abdominal muscles. As soon as the peritoneal cavity is entered, the stylet is withdrawn and the catheter directed to one or other paracolic gutter. The catheter should be stitched in place by a purse-string suture. The catheter exit site should be dressed to prevent infection. 1−2 litre of dialysis fluid is run in, carefully observing any evidence of extravasation. The 'run in' time should be no more than 10 minutes and drain time no more than 20−30 minutes. It is occasionally necessary to run in 1−2 litre with only a marginal return before complete exchanges take place. Any further retention suggests catheter blockage or extravasation. It is advantageous to add heparin (100 u/l) to the first few exchanges to avoid fibrin platelet blockage.

The type and volume of fluid depends on the size of the patient and state of hydration. There are a wide variety of commercially available solutions ranging from a dextrose content of 1.36−6.36%, and sodium concentration of 130−140 mmol/l. Potassium is added as required. Although techniques vary, a cycle time of 10 minutes inflow, 20 minutes equilibration, and 30 minutes outflow, is commonly used. Indications for combinations of varying dextrose and sodium concentrations are shown in Table 4.3.

Table 4.3 Indications for combinations of varying dextrose and sodium concentrations.

Blood volume	Blood pressure	Dextrose concentration (%)	Sodium concentration (mmol/l)
Reduced	Reduced	1.36	140
Normal	Normal	1.36	135
Raised	Normal	3.36–6.36	135
Raised	Raised	3.36–6.36	130

The patient should be encouraged to sit out of bed, take deep breaths and have passive leg movements. Whilst on peritoneal dialysis, a more liberal diet and fluid intake is allowed. Dialysis should continue for at least 48 hours and preferably for no longer than 72 hours. The patient should be weighed at least 4 times a day and blood pressure checked every 4 hours.

Technical complications

• some blood-stained fluid is to be expected occasionally in the first few exchanges
• poor drainage may require either a change in patient posture or the repositioning of the catheter
• leakage of fluid may occur particularly if a tight purse-string suture has not been used
• more serious complications, including extravasation of dialysis fluid or puncture of viscera, are rare

Medical complications

Peritonitis
This is a major complication. It is more likely after a technically poor catheter introduction, poor technique of bag change

after 72 hours of dialysis, or if the catheter is not firmly splinted and adequately dressed. Warning of impending peritonitis may be given by routine culture of dialysis fluid, if an adequate bacteriological back-up service is available. Treatment involves identification and sensitivity testing of the organism and instillation of suitable antimicrobials (see p. 131).

Chest infections
These should be prevented by adequate physiotherapy.

Hypovolaemia
This may occur as a result of over-enthusiastic ultrafiltration. Careful frequent weighing of the patient, regular blood pressure monitoring (including sitting or standing blood pressure) and avoidance of overnight dialysis with osmotically 'strong' (6.36%) dialysis fluid, are factors likely to prevent hypovolaemia, resulting in hypotension, vomiting and, occasionally, diarrhoea. Prompt treatment with plasma and/or saline to raise weight by $1-2$ kg (or whatever is required) is effective.

Disordered electrolyte metabolism
Hyper- and hypokalaemia and -natraemia may be prevented and treated by adjusting the dialysis sodium and potassium levels and oral intake.

Hyperglycaemia
This occasionally occurs if 6.36% glucose dialysate is used for more than 2 or 3 exchanges. Hyperglycaemia may be controlled by *small* doses of subcutaneous insulin (e.g. maximum $8-12$ u $4-6$ hourly), as patients with ARF tend to be very insulin sensitive.

Nitrogen losses
These may be considerable in patients on peritoneal dialysis, amounting up to 20 g per day of protein and amino acids. It is important to counter this loss by encouraging a high-protein diet, (particularly whilst the patient is on dialysis) and to dialyse

for a maximum of 72 hours per week. If a patient requires more dialysis the number of exchanges should be increased, or serious consideration given to haemodialysis.

4.8 Complications of ARF

Pericarditis
A low blood pressure in the face of signs of 'overload', peri-cardial rub, 3rd heart sound or absent apex beat and very soft heart sounds, together with pulsus paradoxus (an inspiratory fall in blood pressure of greater than 10 mmHg) and a rise in JVP with inspiration, all point to pericarditis, usually with effusion. No treatment, other than reducing heparin and con-tinuing dialysis, is usually required, although if tamponade develops, pericardial aspiration may be needed.

Gastro-intestinal bleeding
Bleeding from acute gastric erosions or an acute duodenal ulcer may be prevented by prophylactic antacids such as aluminium hydroxide (20 ml q.d.s).

Disequilibrium
Hypercatabolic patients with high blood urea (> 50 mmol/l) or creatinine (> 2000 µmol/l) concentrations may react adversely (with confusion, tremors and fits) if dialysed with a large surface area dialyser (>1.0 m^2) in the initial few days of dialysis. Short daily dialysis with small surface area dialysers are to be preferred.

Acetate intolerance and lactic acidosis
Acetate intolerance (hypotension, vomiting, headaches) and lactic acidosis, may be prevented by dialysis with bicarbonate dialysate, if haemodialysis is being employed. An increasing number of proportionating machines now have built-in systems for bicarbonate dialysis.

Hypocalcaemia
This is a common complication of acute renal failure and may be severe if secondary to rhabdomyolysis (which is also associ-

ated with disproportionately high creatinine, hyperkalaemia, hyperuricaemia, myoglobinaemia and massive elevation of creatinine phosphokinase (CPK) (>10 000 u/l). In this condition hypocalcaemia may be followed by transient hypercalcaemia in the diuretic phase.

Respiratory complications
These may include pulmonary oedema, infections and, rarely, 'shock lung', requiring ventilation in some patients.

Blood disorders
Anaemia, bleeding tendencies and infections are common.

Total organ failure
Some patients (especially those on intensive care units) present with 'total organ failure' with widespread damage to brain, liver, myocardium, and voluntary muscles. These patients have had either massive trauma, or extensive operations. The prognosis is grave.

4.9 Natural history

The diuretic phase of ARF lasts, on average, 2–3 weeks but may last up to 6 weeks or, rarely, even longer. If recovery is delayed, the patient may have *chronic renal failure* (small kidneys, anaemia on presentation, pigmentation, evidence of erosion on hand films suggestive of hyperparathyroidism), *undiscovered obstruction* (lack of proteinuria, variable urine output) or, rarely, has developed *acute cortical necrosis* (renal cortical calcification on renal biopsy). This latter complication was formerly associated with ARF and obstetric complications, e.g. ante-partum haemorrhage.

During the diuretic phase it is important to keep the weight constant by increasing fluid and electrolyte intake, and providing adequate nutrition.

Most patients with ARF who recover have normal renal function, but up to 20% have variable degrees of renal failure 6–12 months after recovery.

Despite advances in the management of ARF, the often

quoted mortality rate remains unacceptably high, at 50%. This is partly due to the changing causes of ARF, and is distorted by the inclusion of very sick patients with multiple organ problems.

4.10 Prophylaxis

Many patients who develop acute renal failure do so because certain prophylactic measures are not taken.

1 Peri-operative administration of saline to maintain pre-operative weight in patients with existing salt-losing renal failure (e.g. with papillary necrosis). The patient's weight should be carefully monitored.

2 *Careful* use of potent antibiotics, notably aminoglycosides alone or in combination with loop diuretics. Tetracyclines should be avoided in patients with pre-existing renal disease. Diuresis during the administration of cisplatinum and other cytotoxic drugs should be maintained.

3 Avoidance of urography in patients with renal failure associated with diabetes mellitus.

4 Careful screening of renal function and the use of urography in some patients undergoing surgery, e.g. pelvic surgery. The use of mannitol during surgery for obstructive jaundice or extensive organ resection, is debatable but probably justified.

5 Urine culture (or prophylactic antibiotics) before or during instrumentation of the urinary tract.

6 Special care is required in elderly patients undergoing surgery.

7 Careful pre-operative assessment of patients at special risk, including pelvic, biliary and arterial surgery. Obtain pre-operative renal function, avoid dextrose-saline (especially in patients with impaired renal function), and weigh frequently.

8 The administration of i.v. alkali to patients with crush injuries.

9 Call the 'renal team' early.

5: Chronic renal failure (CRF)

5.1 Incidence and causes

It has been independently assessed that approximately 30−50 people aged 15−55 years, per million population, will develop terminal renal failure per year, i.e. approximately 1500−2500 people per year in the UK. If the age range is expanded to include children and adults up to 70 or older the numbers increase to about 70−100 per million per year.

Almost any disease of the kidneys may result in chronic renal failure but the more frequent conditions to do so are shown in the Table 5.1. The percentages refer to patients accepted for dialysis in the UK during 1988.

Note that renal failure especially glomerulonephritis is more common among men than women. Although some patients

Table 5.1 Common and uncommon causes of renal failure.

Common causes	(%)	Uncommon causes	(%)
Glomerulonephritis (with or without histology)	19.3	Myeloma, SLE, Henochs, scleroderma, amyloid, Goodpasture's, HUS	6.0
Pyelonephritis (including reflux nephropathy, stones and obstruction)	13.1	Analgesic nephropathy and other drugs	1.3
Hypertension and renovascular disease	12.1	Congenital and hereditary abnormalities	2.3
Diabetes (type I and II)	12.7	Polyarteritis and Wegener's	1.3
Polycystic kidneys	8.9	Acute tubular necrosis, TB, gout, nephrocalcinosis tumour and trauma	3.5
Unknown	18.9		

Modified from Tufveson *et al.* 1989 *Nephrology Dialysis Transplantation* 4 (suppl. 4). A combined report on regular dialysis and transplantation in Europe XIX 1988.

now have had histologically proven glomerulonephritis, many still present with terminal renal failure, hypertension and bilateral small kidneys. In these patients it is difficult to know whether the hypertension was the cause or result of the renal disease. Renal biopsy in these patients may be difficult and dangerous and the histology reveals 'end-stage' changes compatible with a variety of renal diseases. Features of any particular histological variety of glomerulonephritis may be difficult to determine. Older patients have a higher incidence of diabetes, renovascular disease, obstruction and malignancies as a cause for their renal failure.

5.2 Presentation

Patients with chronic renal failure present in a wide variety of ways. Some patients may be followed for years with gradually worsening renal function, whilst others present with advanced renal failure requiring almost immediate dialysis. The main presenting features include:

- hypertension
- malaise
- gastro-intestinal symptoms
- anaemia
- haematuria
- polyuria

- urinary infections
- renal colic
- pulmonary oedema
- infection
- those of the underlying disease, e.g. diabetes

The lesson to be learned is that renal function should be assessed in any patient with an unexplained illness.

5.3 Clinical features

Symptoms and signs vary from finding virtually nothing abnormal to a severely ill patient with multiple abnormalities. Virtually every system in the body may be involved, including the following:

- cardiovascular (hypertension, ischaemic heart disease, pericarditis)
- respiratory (infection, pulmonary oedema)
- gastro-intestinal (nausea, vomiting, diarrohoea, abdominal

pain, gastro-intestinal haemorrhage, peptic ulcer)
- neurological (neuropathy, tremor, coma, fits, visual deterioration)
- haematological (pallor, petechiae, bruising, frank blood loss),
- locomotor (myopathy, joint pains, arthritis)
- skin (pruritus)
- immunological (liability to infections)
- nephro-urological

5.4 Investigation

The investigation of patients with chronic renal failure should determine the cause of the renal failure, including potentially reversible causes, and act as a baseline for future management. It must include the following examinations in selected patients:
- haematology: full blood count, platelet count, prothrombin time, blood group
- biochemistry: urea, electrolytes, creatinine, creatinine clearance, calcium, phosphate, alkaline phosphatase, liver function tests, urate, 25-OH vitamin D_3, parathyroid hormone, complement, immunoglobulins, urinary protein excretion, protein electrophoresis, Bence-Jones protein
- microbiology: MSU, hepatitis B antigen, HIV antibody status (after counselling)
- radiology: chest, plain abdomen, hands, intravenous urogram (IVU), ultrasound, barium meal, angiography to exclude artery stenosis
- nuclear medicine: renogram, EDTA clearance
- other: electrocardiogram (ECG), occult bloods, gastroscopy (if indicated)

Reversible causes of renal failure include:
- obstruction
- stones
- infection
- electrolyte disturbances, e.g. hypercalcaemia
- drugs, e.g. analgesics, non-steroidal anti-inflammatory drugs
- myeloma

- renovascular diseases, e.g. renal artery stenosis, renal vein thrombosis
- SLE and vasculitis

Management
The art of managing patients with chronic renal failure lies in preventing a decline in renal function and complications. Details of management will be given after a discussion of the main complications of renal failure.

5.5 Complications

The complications of chronic renal failure affect nearly every system of the body. Serious, life-threatening, complications tend to occur with very advanced renal failure (GFR < 4 ml per minute, creatinine concentration of 1200−1500 μmol/l), and should be preventable by dialysis or transplantation.

Cardiovascular complications

Hypertension
This is almost an integral part of the disease process and can hardly be called a complication. Nevertheless, the control of high blood pressure is a key factor in the long-term management of chronic renal failure and depends on the principles outlined in Chapter 11.

Arterial disease
A combination of hypertension, lipid abnormalities and cigarette smoking, increase the incidence of coronary, cerebral and peripheral vascular disease.

Pericarditis
Most patients with renal failure have some degree of fibrinous pericarditis at autopsy. More serious episodes of haemorrhagic pericarditis occur late and are a sign of severe uraemia.

Pulmonary oedema
A combination of fluid overload and a raised left atrial pressure secondary to hypertension may lead to repeated attacks of

pulmonary oedema exacerbated by leaky capillaries and hypo-albuminaemia.

Respiratory complications

Infections are common, including pneumonia and tuberculosis.

Calcium and phosphate metabolism

Chronic renal failure is associated with several distinct disorders of calcium and phosphate metabolism. Some of the main metabolic consequences are outlined in Fig. 5.1.

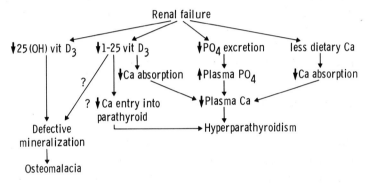

Fig. 5.1 The main metabolic consequences of chronic renal failure.

Hyperparathyroidism

This is the commonest abnormality of calcium metabolism seen in patients with renal failure. Parathyroid hormone levels increase early in renal failure. X-ray changes follow later and symptoms, such as bone pains, fractures and myopathy, present later still. Regular monitoring of serum calcium, phosphate, alkaline phosphatase, and hand X-rays, are important to detect early features of hyperparathyroidism. Elevated parathormone levels may also promote other 'toxic' changes including anaemia, neuropathy and cardiac failure.

Osteomalacia

Osteomalacia (defined histologically) occurs in about 10% of patients with advanced renal failure. The aetiology is controversial, especially the role of 25-OH vitamin D_3 and $1-25$ $(OH)_2$ vitamin D_3 (and other metabolites). Osteomalacia results in bone pain, proximal myopathy and, occasionally, fractures.

A comparison between osteomalacia and hyperparathyroidism is given in Table 5.2.

Table 5.2 A comparison between osteomalacia and hyperparathyroidism.

	Osteomalacia	Hyperparathyroidism
Serum calcium	Reduced ⎤ product low	High or normal ⎤ product high
Serum phosphate	Normal ⎦	High or normal ⎦
Alkaline phosphatase	Increased	Normal or increased
Histology	Increased osteoid, reduced calcification front	Increased osteoclastic activity, tunnelling of cortical bone, increased osteoid
X-ray	Loosers zone	Erosions of hands, clavicle, trochanters; osteosclerosis, vertebral collapse

High calcium and phosphate product
This may induce widespread metastatic and vascular calcification resulting in severe pruritus, red eye and soft-tissue calcification. The treatment of hyperphosphataemia should be a prime aim in the management of patients with chronic renal failure, because not only will it ameliorate metastatic calcification but it may also prevent the development of hyperparathyroidism.

Osteoporosis
This condition (a reduction in absolute amount of bone per unit volume) is also associated with renal failure but is the least understood of the metabolic bone disorders.

Alimentary tract complications

These include peptic ulcers (high gastrin levels), haemorrhagic gastritis or duodenitis (complicated by haematemesis or melaena). Rarely, pancreatitis, peritonitis or diarrhoea, may occur.

Neurological complications

A progressive peripheral neuropathy is a late feature of chronic renal failure preventable by early dialysis or transplantation. Other neurological complications include myoclonic jerks, ('restless legs'), myopathy, fits, drowsiness, and coma.

Joint complications

Gout is surprisingly rare in patients with renal failure, despite elevations in serum urate. High calcium and phosphate products may result in pseudogout or periarticular calcification.

Integument changes

The skin may become thin and dry, subject to infections, and made worse by pruritus. Pigmentation is common. The nails become brittle, ridged and opaque.

Infections

Soft-tissue, respiratory, urinary tract infections and septicaemia are more common, due to suppressed immune responses.

Haematological complications

These include anaemia, a bleeding tendency, gastro-intestinal blood loss, increased red cell breakdown, platelet function abnormalities, and clotting factor deficiencies.

Endocrine changes

- abnormal glucose homeostasis with glucose intolerance and raised circulating levels of pro-insulin
- abnormal thyroid function tests (low T_4, T_3) but normal free T_4, T_3 and normal thyroid-stimulating hormone (TSH) levels, but with abnormal (prolonged) thyroid-releasing hormone (TRH) tests
- abnormal lipid levels, representing type IV hyperlipoproteinaemia
- gonadal abnormalities, including gynaecomastia, low testosterone levels, subfertility, menstrual irregularities, elevated luteinising hormone (LH) and prolactin levels.

5.6 Management of patients with chronic renal failure

The aim of treatment is to:
- maintain renal function as long as possible
- prevent complications
- ease symptoms

All patients may require variations in management from time to time. Most have multiple problems and require careful follow-up with meticulous attention to detail.

Some physicians plot the reciprocal of the plasma creatinine concentration as an index of renal function against time. Acceleration in the decline of the slope suggests that some preventable factor may be present.

Diet

There is now some controlled evidence that lowering the protein intake to 0.5 g of protein/kg body weight per 24 hours, reduces the rate of decline of renal function in patients with renal failure. The diet should be prescribed by a renal dietician. Vitamins and mineral supplements should be given. The phosphate intake should also be reduced.

Some authorities have advocated that an even lower protein intake (0.2 kg protein/kg body weight) avoiding all animal proteins and supplemented by amino or keto acids. However these expensive preparations are not widely available.

The point at which low protein diets are started is debatable but should be in the region of a GFR of 20 ml per minute plasma creatinine approximately 400 μmol/l). Adherence to a low protein diet can be checked by measuring total nitrogen (N) output which is calculated from urea nitrogen (N) excretion and non-N excretion.

$$
\begin{aligned}
\text{Urea N excretion} \quad &= \text{urinary urea mmol per day } (x) \\
&= 2x \text{ mmol N per day} \\
&= 2x \times 0.01258 \text{ g N per day} = A
\end{aligned}
$$

$$
\begin{aligned}
\text{Non-urea N excretion} &= 0.031 \text{ g N/kg per day (constant)} \\
&= B
\end{aligned}
$$

$$
\begin{aligned}
\text{Total N excretion} \quad &= A + B \text{ (g N) per day} \\
&= A + B \times 6.25 \text{ g protein per day}
\end{aligned}
$$

This should correspond to the intake, providing that the patient is in a steady state and in nitrogen balance.

A raised uric acid is a common finding in patients with chronic renal failure. Hyperuricaemia rarely results in clinical gout or other adverse effects, and there appears to be little gained from giving routine allopurinol.

Fat and carbohydrate content
Sufficient calories (2000–3000 per day) should be given to prevent loss in body weight. At one time, high-fat diets were recommended but the recognition of abnormal fat metabolism has resulted in a more prudent approach. Simple reductions in saturated fatty acids and high carbohydrate foods may be sufficient to reverse abnormal hyperlipoprotein pattern. Drugs such as clofibrate should be used with extreme caution.

Salt and water balance and control of hypertension

Lack of salt and water has a profound adverse effect on kidney function and may be caused by anorexia with inadequate intake, diarrhoea and vomiting, or enforced dehydration prior to such investigations as urography, barium enema, or when the patient

Table 5.3 Summary of treatment of chronic renal failure.

Clinical or biochemical abnormality	Indications	Treatment
Nitrogen retention	GFR <20 ml per minute	Diet 0.5 g protein/kg per 24 hours, low phosphates and supplemental vitamins
Salt and water balance	Sodium depletion	Saline, Slow sodium, sodium bicarbonate
	Sodium excess	Frusemide, bumetanide (in high doses), reduce sodium intake
Potassium balance	Hyperkalaemia	(see p. 32)
	Hypokalaemia	Slow-release potassium chloride
Acidosis	pH <7.2 bicarbonate <15 mmol/l	Sodium bicarbonate tablets
Hypertension		Propranolol, metoprolol, vasodilators, Ca channel blockers, angiotension converting enzyme inhibitors, diuretics (rarely)
Calcium and phosphate metabolism	PO_4 >2.5 mmol/l	Dietary reduction, Aludrox, calcium carbonate
	Ca <2.0 mmol/l	Calcium carbonate, cholecalciferol, calcitriol or alfacalcidol
	Ca >2.7 mmol/l	Reduce calcium and vitamin D intake or parathyroidectomy if hypercalcaemia persists
Urate metabolism	Gout	Allopurinol
Restless legs		Clonazepam
Pruritus		Chlorpheniramine, aluminium hydroxide, emulsifying ointment
Hyperlipidaemia		Diet

For further details of prescribing in chronic renal failure see Chapter 12.

is subject to a general anaesthetic. Certain patients are at a special risk including those with long-standing obstruction, reflux nephropathy, papillary necrosis and medullary cystic disease. In all these situations a vicious cycle is set up (Fig. 5.2).

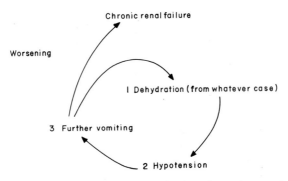

Fig. 5.2 Continuous cycle caused by the lack of salt and water in the kidney.

This cycle can only be broken by rehydration and treatment of the initial cause of dehydration. The *key* to correct management lies in accurate *weighing* of the patient at all times. Some patients require supplementary sodium either as slow sodium (10 mmol per tablet) or sodium bicarbonate (600 mg $\equiv$ 4.8 mmol per tablet).

As renal function declines, sodium excretion falls and the patient may pass from sodium loss to sodium retention. This calls for the utmost vigilance in monitoring correct salt and water balance and blood pressure. An occasional patient will need both hypotensive agents and sodium supplements to optimize renal function and blood pressure.

Hypertension
Adequate control of hypertension is an important factor in the maintenance of renal function. The causes of hypertension are described in detail in Chapter 11. Although in theory there is a balance between volume factors and plasma renin activity, in practice control of the blood pressure in patients with chronic

renal failure requires the use of hypotensive drugs rather than volume-depletion measures. Standard therapy includes the use of a β-blocker with or without a vasodilator. The choice of which β-blocker or vasodilator is a personal one. Certain β-blockers (e.g. propranolol) may impair renal blood flow in patients with advanced renal failure whilst others, (e.g. atenolol) require smaller doses as the drug is excreted unchanged in the urine (Chapter 12). Of the vasodilator drugs, hydralazine in doses above 200 mg per day may cause an illness like systemic lupus erythematosus (SLE) and prazosin should be used with caution since there is increased sensitivity to its hypotensive effect. Currently metoprolol (b.d. or t.d.s.) or atenalol (o.d.) supplemented by nifedipine (b.d.) are widely used. The place of angiotension connecting enzyme (ACE) inhibitors is under assessment in patients with renal failure. Deterioration of renal function in patients given ACE inhibitors strongly suggests renovascular disease as the cause of renal failure.

Patients with chronic renal failure occasionally develop *malignant hypertension*. The treatment of this condition is discussed in Chapter 11.

Potassium and acid-base balance

Hyperkalaemia tends to occur late (GFR < 10 ml per minute) in patients with chronic renal failure, unless precipitated by potassium sparing diuretics, (spironolactone, amiloride, or triamterene), severe acidosis, or an intercurrent infection. Nevertheless, constant vigilance is mandatory and dietary advice, and occasional use of resins, may be required. Unexplained hyperkalaemia may be due to low renin levels with hypoaldosteronism, a rare condition in older patients with mild renal failure, especially associated with diabetes or obstruction. Treatment is by relieving obstruction and by the judicious use of fludrocortisone (0.1−0.5 mg per day).

Although most patients with advanced renal failure have compensated acidosis (low serum bicarbonate), very few have acidaemia. Acute changes in renal function or terminal renal failure may result in severe acidosis, requiring treatment with sodium bicarbonate by mouth or intravenously.

Calcium and phosphate balance

Control of *hyperphosphataemia* results in a reduction in hyper-parathyroidism and metastatic calcification. Control may be achieved by either dietary means (Appendix 6) or the use of aluminium hydroxide such as Aludrox (30 ml t.d.s.), Alu-Cap (3 t.d.s.) or Aludrox tabs (3 t.d.s.). *Hypocalcaemia* may be corrected by giving calcium carbonate either as a mixture (e.g. 1 g of calcium carbonate in 5 ml) as Titralac tablets ($CaCO_3$ 420 mg per tablet) or Calcichew (1260 mg $CaCO_3$ per tablet). Up to 15 g of calcium carbonate or 6 or more Titralac tablets may be required. Calcium carbonate also blocks some absorption of phosphate and corrects metabolic acidosis. Frequent monitoring of serum calcium is required. Deficiency in $1-25$ $(OH)_2$ vitamin D_3 has prompted the use of either 1-α vitamin D_3 (alfacalcidol) or $1-25$ $(OH)_2$ vitamin D_3 (calcitriol) to correct the various skeletal abnormalities. The results have not been an unqualified success since the dose required to suppress hyperparathyroidism may be close to the dose which produces hypercalcaemia. Furthermore, both meta-bolites may potentiate the absorption of phosphate, which counteracts the anti-parathormone activity and may result in high calcium and phosphate products. Both have been used in the treatment of osteomalacia and, after parathyroidectomy, to correct hypocalcaemia. Both are preferable to long-acting preparations of vitamin D or synthetic analogues (calciferol or dihydrotachysterol) which have to be given in large doses and whose side-effects (hypercalcaemia) may last for weeks or even months after withdrawal of the drug. Deficiency of 25 OH vitamin D_3 should be corrected by the administration of chole-calciferol 250 mg daily or on alternate days; or Calcium with vitamin D tablets (BNF), one daily.

Hyperuricaemia

It is unlikely that minor elevations ($0.4-0.6$ mmol/l or $6-8$ mg per 100 ml) of the plasma urate will result in either gout or worsening renal function. If gout develops allopurinol may be used.

Dosage
- allopurinol 100 mg daily if GFR < 10 ml per minute
- allopurinol 200 mg daily if GFR 10−50 ml per minute

Infection

All infections should be promptly treated. Unexplained pyrexia, particularly in Asian patients, may indicate tuberculosis which may be pulmonary, abdominal, hepatic, bony or confined to the urinary tract.

Drug therapy

All drugs must be carefully monitored, avoiding nephrotoxic drugs including tetracyclines and aminoglycosides. Some drugs contain sodium (e.g. carbenicillin) or potassium (e.g. phenethicillin). Drug therapy of all kinds is discussed in detail in Chapter 12.

5.8 Conclusion

Treatment of 'end-stage' renal disease (GFR < 5 ml per minute)

At some stage discussion about the future with the patient and relatives should take place. This is never easy. If dialysis is likely, a fistula should be created 2−3 months before dialysis is commenced.

The choice between haemodialysis, peritoneal dialysis and transplantation is discussed in Chapter 7.

Discussion is best conducted in a centre with a renal unit, and including a social worker, dialysis nursing staff and physician.

One final word — a plea

Do not delay in sending patients to renal units until immediate dialysis is required. Various medical and social issues may have to be discussed at an earlier stage. Furthermore, severely uraemic patients (creatinine > 1200 mmol/l, GFR > 4 mol per minute may have life-threatening complications, and rehabilitation is greatly prolonged once dialysis is started.

Do not discuss dialysis until a renal unit has accepted a patient for dialysis or transplantation.

Do not 'cut down' over veins which may have to be used for fistulae or shunts.

6: Haematuria, proteinuria and glomerulonephritis

6.1 Haematuria
(>10 red blood cells (RBC)/mm^3)

Haematuria is an important indicator of nephro-urological disease. Frank blood, clots, and heavy macroscopic haematuria, clearing as micturition proceeds, are more likely to be associated with bladder problems. 'Smoky' urine, microscopic haematuria, with proteinuria and loin pain, suggest renal disease. A guide towards the investigation of haematuria is given in Table 6.1.

Table 6.1 Investigation of haematuria.

Cause	Investigation
'Pseudo' haematuria vaginal bleeding	Careful history and physical examination; careful collection of MSU
Bladder pathology polyps stones tumour infection	Urine culture, urine cytology, IVU, cystocopy
Renal pathology stones papillary necrosis tumours polycystic disease glomerulonephritis renal infarcts loin pain and haematuria syndrome	IVU, arteriogram, ultrasound, cystoscopy, renal biopsy
bleeding diathesis 'march' haematuria	Full clotting screen

The following points concerning haematuria without proteinuria are worth noting:

- acute bacterial cystitis is commonly associated with haematuria
- cystitis, tumours and stones are the commonest causes of haematuria
- cystoscopy usually precedes renal biopsy even in younger patients in the search for haematuria
- arteriography, if indicated, precedes renal biopsy
- haematuria occurring during anticoagulation may indicate occult disease and investigation is justified
- renal pelvic tumours are notoriously difficult to diagnose and require careful radiological assessment, including tomography, retrograde urograms and cytology
- exercise potentiates bleeding due to glomerulonephritis as well as revealing other lesions, e.g. 'march' haematuria

Some patients, (especially young men) can continue to have episodes of severe haematuria despite intensive investigation. They may suffer from small leaking arteriovenous (A−V) malformations beyond the resolution of conventional investigational procedures. They may respond to tranexamic acid (500 mg q.d.s.) although great care has to be taken to avoid clot colic. Tranexamic acid is best avoided in patients with renal failure. A summary of investigation of red urine is given in Fig. 6.1.

6.2 Proteinuria

Normal adults excrete up to 200 mg of protein per day, mainly as mucoprotein from the kidney and bladder. Protein excretion in excess of this is abnormal. Transient, and usually trivial, proteinuria is not uncommonly found in hospital practice and may be due to exercise, fevers, intercurrent infections, operations, hypothermia and blood transfusions.

Asymptomatic proteinuria

This is an important finding with varying clinical significance which may relate to life insurance and employment prospects. Unnecessary alarm may be caused unless the following points are remembered.

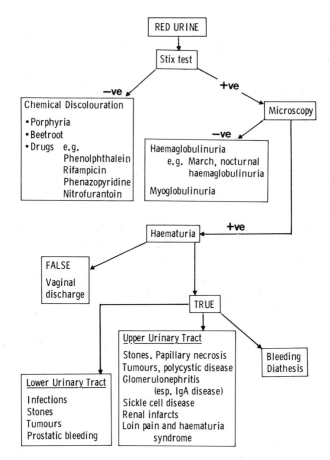

Fig. 6.1 Investigation of red urine.

1 'Stix' tests are very sensitive and detect normal amounts of protein in concentrated urines (as little as 40 mg/l).
2 If proteinuria is found it must be confirmed on clean-catch, mid-stream, early morning urine specimens, preferably on two or three occasions, using 25% salicylsulphonic acid.
3 25% salicylsulphonic acid is less sensitive than 'Stix' tests, detecting protein concentration down to 300 mg/l; it detects Bence-Jones protein but may give false-positive results in patients taking penicillins, tolbutamide or following X-ray contrast media.

Orthostatic

In young people, proteinuria may be orthostatic and is confirmed by comparing post-ambulatory and post-supine overnight urine samples. Orthostatic proteinuria carries an excellent prognosis and both patient and parent can be reassured.

Glomerular

As a rough guide, glomerular proteinuria usually exceeds 1 g per day and proteinuria associated with the nephrotic syndrome usually exceeds 3.0 g per day/1.73 m^2 body surface area.

Tubular

Tubular proteinuria is present in a concentration of between 0.8 and 1.0 g per 24 hours. The causes include:

- aminoacidurias (Fanconi's syndrome)
- heavy metal poisoning (e.g. Cd)
- inflammatory diseases, e.g. sarcoidosis, infections
- congenital abnormalities (e.g. cystic disease of the medulla)
- obstruction

Tubular proteinuria is 'non-selective' (see below), and may be confirmed by defining the underlying abnormality or using the β_2-microglobulin test (p. 13).

Protein selectivity

This term is used to describe the fact that in some renal diseases smaller molecular weight proteins are lost in the urine, whereas higher molecular weight proteins are not. Formerly, the clearance of IgG was compared to the clearance of albumin, but transferrin is now often used. Since the urine volumes are the same,

$$\% \text{ protein selectivity} = \frac{\text{clearance IgG}}{\text{clearance transferrin}} \times 100$$

$$= \frac{\text{UIgG}}{\text{PIgG}} \bigg/ \frac{\text{Utrans}}{\text{Ptrans}} \times 100$$

where UIgG is urinary IgG, PIgG plasma IgG, Utrans urinary transferrin, and Ptrans plasma transferrin, in any randomly collected urine sample. Highly selective proteinuria ($< 10\%$ or selectivity index of <0.1) is found in minimal change GN and early diabetic glomerulosclerosis, moderately selective proteinuria (10−30% or selectivity index 0.1−0.3), in most other forms of glomerulonephritis, and non-selective proteinuria ((>30%) or selectivity index >0.3) in GN and tubular proteinuria.

Persistent non-orthostatic proteinuria
This requires further investigation with some or all of the following tests, depending on the clinical features. The investigations in parentheses are rarely required.
• haematological: FBC, erythrocyte sedimentation rate and clotting screen
• biochemical: urea, electrolytes, liver function tests, serum proteins, protein electrophoresis, creatinine clearance, 24-hour urinary protein excretion, (protein selectivity), (urinary protein electrophoresis), (Bence-Jones protein), and (glucose tolerance test)
• serological: ASO titre, ANF, DNA titre, immunoglobulins, complement, hepatitis B antigen, (immune complexes)
• X-ray: IVU, (arteriogram), ultrasound
• microbiology: throat swab, MSU, (blood cultures)
• renal biopsy
   A summary of investigation of proteinuria is given in Fig. 6.2.

6.3 Glomerulonephritis, nephritic and nephrotic syndromes

The term 'glomerulonephritis' (GN) should be reserved for histological appearances, since the correlation between what is found histologically and clinically is at best tenuous. 'Nephritis' should be avoided, and although 'nephritic syndrome' and 'nephrotic syndrome' have little to commend them they are well-accepted terms.

Relation between histology and clinical findings

Patients with different histological forms of glomerulonephritis present with a variety of clinical features, and attempts to

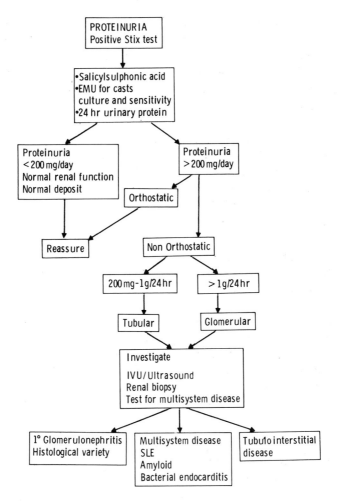

Fig. 6.2 Investigation of proteinuria.

relate any one clinical presentation with a single histological appearance are impossible. Nevertheless, certain histological types are associated with the specific clinical features summarized in Table 6.2.

Aetiology and pathogenesis of glomerulonephritis

The precise aetiology responsible for the majority of patients with various forms of glomerulonephritis remains unknown.

Table 6.2 Histological types and clinical features of GN.

Histology of GN	Usual presentation	Unusual presentation
Acute (exudative)	Nephritic syndrome	Proteinuria nephrotic syndrome, renal failure
Minimal change	Nephrotic syndrome	Proteinuria
Focal sclerosis	Nephrotic syndrome, proteinuria	Renal failure
Focal and segmental	Haematuria, nephrotic syndrome, proteinuria	Renal failure
Mesangio-proliferative	Proteinuria haematuria	Renal failure
Membranous	Nephrotic syndrome, proteinuria	Renal failure
Mesangio-capillary	Nephrotic syndrome, proteinuria, haematuria	Renal failure
Rapidly progressive	Renal failure	Proteinuria, nephrotic syndrome
End-stage	Renal failure	

There are undoubted geographical variations in the incidence and variety of glomerulonephritides. Abnormal host factors, such as tissues types and complement abnormalities, may predispose certain individuals to develop glomerulonephritis. Traditionally, glomerular damage may be produced by the following.

Immune complex disease
(> 95% of all patients with glomerulonephritis)

This occurs when circulating immune complexes are thought to be passively trapped in the glomerulus and elicit an inflammatory response through the mediation of complement and other inflammatory mechanisms. Immune complexes are deposited along the capillary basement membrane or within the mesangium in a *granular* pattern. The list of responsible antigens is long and in many instances anecdotal, but the more common agents include:

- nephritogenic strains of streptococci, leading to acute glomerulonephritis
- drugs (gold, penicillamine), infections (malaria, schistosomiasis), endogenous antigen (tumours, thyroglobulin), all leading to membranous glomerulonephritis
- staphylococcus albus (shunt nephritis), leading to mesangiocapillary glomerulonephritis
- DNA (SLE), leading to various histological forms

This list is deliberately short but shows the variety of exogenous and endogenous agents responsible. It must be stressed that in the majority of patients with deposits of immune complexes, no aetiological agent is discernable.

Anti glomerular basement membrane (GBM)
(< 5% of all patients with glomerulonephritis)

This condition occurs when circulating immunoglobulins directed against glomerular and lung capillary basement membrane elicit an inflammatory response. The deposition of immunoglobulin is *linear* along the glomerular capillary basement membrane.

The traditional understanding has been challenged in clinical practice and experimentally. Anti-GBM antibodies may be a secondary rather than a primary event, or secondary to GBM altered by a variety of stimuli. Further, circulating immune complexes found readily in acute glomerulonephritis are unusual in membranous glomerulonephritis. Thus the focus has switched to studying formations of immune complexes and inflammatory responses within the glomerulus, and identifying abnormalities in each variety of histological abnormality described.

Acute nephritic syndrome
(acute glomerulonephritis, acute nephritis)

This syndrome is characterized by proteinuria, haematuria, hypertension and salt and water retention. The most common histological association is proliferative glomerulonephritis but other histological abnormalities, notably focal and segmental glomerulonephritis, mesangio-capillary glomerulonephritis and polyarteritis nodosa, occasionally present in this way.

Acute proliferative glomerulonephritis often follows an infection with a nephritogenic strain of β-haemolytic streptococcus (Lancefield Type A, groups 4 and 12), usually with tonsillitis, but occasionally after skin sepsis. 1−2 weeks after the initial infection the patient notices dependent and non-dependent oedema, oliguria and smoky urine. Clinical examination reveals hypertension, oedema and a rise in JVP. Proteinuria, haematuria and granular casts are found. A throat swab may show haemolytic streptococci and the ASO titre is raised. Many cases are mild with normal renal function; rarely, renal failure, severe hypertension and pulmonary oedema develops. Renal biopsy findings are shown in Table 6.3.

The disease is usually self-limiting, requiring only rest, sodium restriction, penicillin and, rarely, a diuretic or hypotensive drug. The prognosis is excellent, especially in children. It is doubtful whether long-term penicillin is required but this is customarily given. Occasionally, patients with acute glomerulonephritis develop rapidly progressive glomerulonephritis with glomerular crescents and worsening renal function (see p. 88). Proteinuria may persist following acute glomerulonephritis for months or even years. The prognosis may be guarded for patients with persistent protein in excess of 0.3 g per 24 hours.

Nephrotic syndrome

Nephrotic syndrome consists of the classical triad of proteinuria, hypoalbuminaemia and oedema. There is only a loose relationship between the levels of proteinuria, serum albumin and oedema. Young patients may have heavy proteinuria and an albumin of 20 g/l without oedema, whereas older patients may develop oedema at albumin levels of 30 g/l. The difference lies in the efficiency of the lymphatics. The levels of proteinuria and serum albumin are also only roughly related.

Other features include increased plasma α_2- and β-globulins, hypercholesterolaemia, hypercoagulation, loss of binding proteins (e.g. transferrin, vitamin D binding protein), and reduction in binding sites on albumin for certain drugs, e.g. clofibrate.

Pathogenesis
Although the lower serum oncotic pressure undoubtedly promotes the formation of oedema, the cause of the sodium retention is unknown. It is not related to renin, angiotensin or aldosterone levels, but is probably due to intra-renal physical factors.

Treatment
Many patients with nephrotic syndrome have renal lesions for which there is no specific treatment. Treatment is therefore symptomatic and supporting measures include the following.

1 Normal protein intake, providing that renal function is normal. The maximum synthetic rate of albumin is increased in the nephrotic syndrome but this does not match the maximum catabolic rate since serum albumin is low.

2 Dietary cholesterol and saturated fats should be reduced. It is best to avoid clofibrate and other lipid-lowering agents.

3 Vitamin supplements including 25-OH vitamin D_3 or 1-25 $(OH)_2$ vitamin D_3 may be given if the level of 25-OH vitamin D_3 is less than 15 mmol/l.

4 Exercise is to be encouraged. Prophylactic anticoagulation should be given to cover major operations. Full anticoagulation is required for thrombotic episodes.

Diuretics are widely used in the management of nephrotic syndrome, but should be used with caution.

• loop diuretics (frusemide, bumetanide) are more effective than thiazide diuretics

• large doses may have to be given (e.g. up to 1 g of frusemide per day)

• loop diuretics may be combined with potassium sparing diuretics such as amiloride, triamterene or spironolactone, providing that renal function is normal

• beware of inducing hypovolaemia with hypotension and

worsening renal function. This is a particular problem *in children.*

• if the patient has gross oedema or hypovolaemia, or if the oedema is 'diuretic resistant', an infusion of salt-free albumin combined with a slow i.v. infusion of frusemide (250 mg) and aminophylline (250 mg) is often effective in producing a diuresis, which, once started, may continue with diuretics alone

• careful monitoring of weight, blood pressure (lying and standing) and electrolytes, is mandatory at all times

• if treatment with large doses of frusemide fail, it is worth trying metolazone, a powerful thiazide diuretic, since many cases of refractory oedema respond to this drug

Patients with nephrotic syndrome are susceptible to infections of all types.

6.4 Types of glomerulonephritis

Glomerulonephritis can present as asymptomatic proteinuria, haematuria, nephrotic syndrome, hypertension, renal failure, or as part of a generalized disease such as SLE, diabetes, amyloid or polyarteritis. Men tend to be affected more often than women in all the histological varieties. Although the correlation between histology and clinical findings is, as previously stated, poor, the different types of glomerulonephritis are best discussed under histological headings. Further details are given in Table 6.3.

Minimal change glomerulonephritis

This is associated with the nephrotic syndrome, in children, adolescents and, occasionally, adults. Proteinuria may be massive — up to 20 g per day. Serum albumin may be 20 g/l or less. Renal function is usually normal, haematuria is rare. The aetiology is unknown, some patients have a history of atopy; very rarely, minimal change glomerulonephritis is associated with reticuloses or other neoplasms.

Table 6.3 Summary of biopsy findings.

Condition	Light microscopy	Immunofluorescence	Electron microscopy
Acute post-streptococcal GN	Glomerular cellular proliferation (exudative), polymorphs, interstitial infiltrate	Widespread granular deposits of IgG, IgM and C3 on capillary walls	Prominent extra-membranous 'humps'
Nil or minimal change	Glomeruli normal, tubules, lipid-containing cells	Nil, very occasional mesangial deposit of IgM	Foot process fusion
Focal sclerosis (focal hyalinosis)	Focal glomerulosclerosis starting in juxta medullary glomeruli	IgM in sclerosed areas	Foot process fusion
Focal and segmental GN	Slight increase in mesangial matrix and cellularity, occasional adhesions	Mesangial IgA deposits, occasional IgG and C3	Mesangial electron dense deposits
Henoch-Schönlein purpura	Slight increase in mesangial matrix and cellularity occasionally proliferative with crescents	Mesangial IgA, IgG, C3 and fibrinogen	Mesangial electron dense deposits
Mesangio-proliferative GN	Increase in mesangial cell nuclei	Variable deposition of IgA, IgM in mesangial regions	Variable mesangial electron dense deposits
Membranous GN ('epimembranous')	'Thickened' capillary wall, no proliferation	Capillary wall granular deposit of IgG, C3, occasionally IgA	Subepithelial discrete deposits
Mesangio-capillary GN ('membrano-proliferative lobular')	Mesangial matrix ↑, mesangial cell proliferation, tramline basement membranes	Type 1: C3, Type 2: IgG, IgM, C3 on capillary walls and mesangium	1 Dense linear deposit along basement membranes 2 Widespread subendothelial deposits
Rapidly progressive GN ('extra-capillary GN')	Marked proliferation including crescents, vasculitis, tubulo-interstitial changes	Variable granular or linear capillary wall staining with IgG, C3, occasionally IgM, IgA; fibrin in crescents	Great variation depending on light microscopy
End-stage	Variable glomerular obsolescence, marked tubulo-interstitial disease	Variable	Great variation depending on light microscopy

↑ Increase

Treatment

Steroids have been used traditionally in both children and adults. Prednisolone, 2 mg/kg in children and 60 mg daily in adults (preferably on alternate days), is given for 6 weeks. A diuresis usually takes place within 2–3 weeks. Once remission has occurred, the steroid dosage is lowered and gradually tapered off over 3–4 weeks. Steroids should not be given for longer than 6–8 weeks. Approximately 70% of patients will respond to steroids, however 50% will relapse within 1–2 years.

Patients who relapse frequently ('steroid-dependent') may be given cyclophosphamide (2 mg/kg dose adjustments according to the white blood cell count) for 4–6 weeks under steroid cover. Approximately 60% of patients will respond to this treatment; those who do not, or those who fail to respond to steroids in the first place probably suffer with focal glomerulosclerosis. Cyclophosphamide may cause alopecia (temporary, but the patient may require a wig), bone-marrow depression and haemorrhagic cystitis. In the long term, gonadal dysfunction may result and the risks should be explained to the patient, or parents. Long-term treatment with steroids in children, even on an alternate day basis, should be avoided because of growth problems. An alternative approach to cyclophophamide is to use cyclosporin 4–8 mg/kg which has been found to be effective in some cases of steroid dependent minimal change GN.

Focal and segmental glomerulosclerosis (FSGS)

Diagnosis of this condition tends to be 'by exclusion'. Classically, the lesion affects the juxta medullary glomeruli and may be missed in biopsies confined to cortical tissue. Focal glomerulosclerosis presents as the nephrotic syndrome, or occasionally as proteinuria or renal failure. It is occasionally associated with diabetes, hypertension, reflux nephropathy, heroin addiction and HIV infection. The pathogenesis is unknown. Up to 30% of patients with idiopathic FSGS may respond to steroids and a few extra to cyclosporin. Other immunosuppressive drugs are of no proven value. The disease may recur in transplanted kidneys.

Focal and segmental glomerulonephritis ('focal nephritis')

This presents mainly as recurrent attacks of haematuria but also, rarely, as proteinuria, nephrotic syndrome or renal failure. The outstanding histological feature is messangial deposits of IgA described by Berger ('IgA disease' or even 'Berger's disease') usually with complement and IgG. Serum complement, IgG and IgM levels are normal, but IgA levels may be raised.

Focal and segmental glomerulonephritis is the commonest histological variety of glomerulonephritis, accounting for 14% of all biopsies in the British Medical Research Council (MRC) registry. No treatment is necessary, but follow-up is required since some patients, particularly those with nephrotic syndrome or mild renal failure on presentation, may suffer further renal damage. Focal and segmental glomerulonephritis may recur in transplanted kidneys.

Henoch−Schönlein disease

Although strictly a multisystem disease, Henoch−Schönlein purpura resembles focal and segmental glomerulonephritis histologically and will be considered here. Not all patients suffer the classical triad of purpura, abdominal pain and arthralgia, and many do not have proteinuria or haematuria. Renal failure is rare and is usually associated with crescents on biopsy. The histology resembles focal, segmental, glomerulonephritis except that mesangial fibrinogen is present.

Generally, children have a better prognosis than adults. Steroids and immunosuppressive drugs have been given to patients with worsening renal function but there is no controlled trial to evaluate their effectiveness.

Mesangio-proliferative glomerulonephritis

This is a histological entity with a variety of clinical presentations, including asymptomatic proteinuria, haematuria and nephrotic syndrome. There is some overlap with focal and segmental glomerulonephritis, including patients with IgA mesangial deposits. It is possible that some patients represent early forms of mesangio-capillary glomerulonephritis.

Membranous ('epimembranous') glomerulonephritis

This condition presents mainly as proteinuria or nephrotic syndrome. Light microscopy shows thick renal capillary walls formerly thought to be widened basement membranes (hence 'membranous'), but now known to be due to subepithelial electron-dense deposits, with growth of new basement membrane between deposits. Renal function on presentation is usually normal, as are immunoglobulins and complement.

Aetiology
In contrast to other types, membranous glomerulonephritis is associated with certain well-defined diseases:
- infections: e.g. malaria, leprosy, schistosomiasis, hepatitis B, syphilis, and Epstein–Barr infections
- neoplasms: colon, stomach, pancreas, lung, lymphomas
- endogenous antigen: thyroglobulin, DNA
- drugs, e.g. gold, penicillamine, tridione, probenecid, and tolbutamide

Evidence of circulating immune complexes is meagre in membranous glomerulonephritis. Subepithelial electron-dense deposits may consist of locally complexed immunoglobulins (e.g. IgG/anti-IgG complexes).

Treatment
Treatment of infections, withdrawal of drugs and, possibly, reduction in tumour mass, may be followed by reduction of proteinuria and remission of the disease. Most causes, however, have no obvious associated antigen ('idiopathic membranous glomerulonephritis'). Early trials suggested that prednisolone 125 mg on alternate days, for 6 weeks may reduce the chances of the patient developing renal failure, but this has not been confirmed by a British MRC trial. There is some evidence that worsening renal function in a patient with membranous glomerulonephritis may respond to alternating 4 weekly courses of steroids and chlorambucil. The steroids are

given as methylprednisolone 1.0 g i.v., three doses daily, followed by prednisolone for a further 25 days. Chlorambucal is then commenced at 0.2 mg/kg (reducing the dose if marrow toxicity results) for 28 days. This is followed by further alternating monthly courses of steroids and chlorambucil.

Renal vein thrombosis

This occasionally complicates membranous glomerulonephritis and should be excluded if there is unexplained worsening of renal function or nephrotic syndrome or if a pulmonary embolus occurs.

Mesangio-capillary glomerulonephritis

This condition is characterized by an increase in mesangial matrix which appears to split the capillary basement membranes and is divided into two types.

Type 1. Patients with subendothelial deposits with complement deficiency activated by the 'classical' pathway (low C3, C4, C2 and C1).

Type 2. Patients with 'dense deposit' disease apparent on electron-microscopy, with mesangial cell proliferation, negative staining for immunoglobulins, and positive for C3. Complement is activated by the alternate pathway with low C3 but normal C4, C2 and C1. A circulating factor which activates C3 *in vitro* has been described (C3 Ne_f). Some patients have partial lipodystrophy.

In both types, patients present with nephrotic syndrome, proteinuria (nearly always with haematuria) or acute nephritic syndrome. Some patients have unexplained anaemia. Treatment is symptomatic only (see nephrotic syndrome). The use of immunosuppressive drugs is empirical. Some trials have recommended the use of steroids and anti-platelet drugs whereas others have not supported this approach. More information is needed before patients are treated with drugs which carry unacceptable side-effects.

Rapidly progressive glomerulonephritis (RPGN)

This is not a single disease, nor a single histological entity but comprises a group of patients who show a rapid reduction in renal function and a proliferative (extra-capillary) glomerulonephritis, usually with crescent formation. A number of different diseases may produce this histological entity including: post-streptococcal glomerulonephritis, vasculitis (polyarteritis, Wegener's granulomatosis), Henoch–Schönlein purpura (p. 85), SLE (p. 90), bacterial endocarditis (p. 94), and Goodpasture's syndrome (see below). Differentiation between the various causes of rapidly progressive glomerulonephritis is made by both clinical and histological assessment. Immunofluorescence may show:

- granular deposits of immunoglobulin and complement (post-streptococcal), usually with fibrinogen in crescents
- linear deposits of IgG along the capillary wall (Goodpasture's syndrome)
- no deposits of immunoglobulin
- vasculitic lesions

Goodpasture's syndrome

Goodpasture's syndrome consists of a flu-like illness often in young men with haemoptysis, anaemia, proteinuria and bilateral pulmonary opacities on chest X-ray. Lung function shows an increased transfer factor. Circulating anti-GBM antibodies are found. Renal function may show rapid deterioration.

Prognosis and treatment

Speed of assessment is mandatory in the management of patients with RPGN. A renal biopsy showing > 70% of glomeruli with crescents indicates a bad prognosis. Anti-GBM antibodies (to confirm Goodpastures disease) and anti-neutrophil cytoplasmic antibodies (to confirm Wegener's or microscopic polyarteritis) are essential. The management may be summarized in Table 6.4.

Table 6.4 Management of rapidly progressive glomerulonephritis (RPGN).

	Goodpastures	Wegener's or microscopic vasculitis	Other histological varieties
Non-dialysis dependent patients	Steroids, cytotoxic agents, plasmaphoresis	Steroids, cyclophosphamide, plasma phoresis (?)	Steroids, cytotoxic antiplatelet drugs, plasma phoresis
Dialysis dependent patients	As above, but less successful	Steroids, cyclophosphamide, plasma phoresis	All tried and unproven

End-stage glomerulonephritis

Many patients do not present with glomerulonephritis until they have advanced uraemia. The kidneys are small and difficult (occasionally dangerous) to biopsy. Histology reveals variable glomerular abnormalities, marked tubulo-interstitial inflammation, and vascular changes. Biopsy may be attempted to reveal unusual histological features such as Fabry's disease (p. 169) or to try and exclude renal disease likely to be transmitted to a transplanted kidney (focal sclerosis, focal and segmental glomerulonephritis, mesangio-capillary glomerulonephritis, (dense deposit variety), or amyloidosis). It must be remembered that the natural history of some forms of glomerulonephritis may be longer than the natural history of the renal transplant.

Glomerular and tubular damage

Glomerulonephritis is acknowledged to be the commonest cause of chronic renal failure in both sexes but there is a tendency to ignore tubular damage. Although some tubular damage may be secondary to vascular changes, most is of uncertain aetiology and may be of greater significance in renal impairment than glomerular abnormalities.

Comparative prognoses
Sufficient evidence is now available for long-term prognoses to be plotted by the life table method. This shows that histological entities have distinct natural histories and gives baselines upon which future therapies should be judged (Fig. 6.3).

6.5 Secondary glomerulonephritis

The kidney in systemic lupus erythematosus (SLE)

Systemic lupus erythematosus (SLE) is an important, although rare, cause of renal failure, at least in Europe. Virtually all types of histological changes have been found in patients with

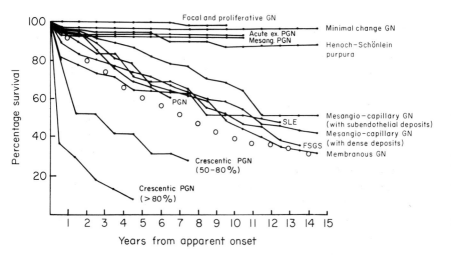

Fig. 6.3 Long-term prognosis plotted by the life table method. Survival of various histological types of GN involving over 2500 patients adequately characterized at onset. For comparison, survival dates for stage 1 and 2 carcinoma of the breast are given. Acute ex. PGN: acute exudative proliferative GN; Mesang. PGN: mesangio-proliferative GN; SLE: systemic lupus erythematosus; FSGS: focal segmental glomerulosclerosis; Crescentic PGN: proliferative GN with crescents. (○○○) Stage 1 and 2 carcinoma of breast (Brinley and Haybittle (1975) *Lancet* ii, 95).

SLE, including no change, focal, membranous and diffuse proliferative changes, with and without crescents. In general (although this is still under study), the prognosis is rather better for focal and membranous lesions as compared to proliferative glomerulonephritis (especially with subendothelial deposits).

Patients, usually female, present with features of SLE (fever, arthritis, rashes, leucopenia, raised ESR, positive ANF, positive DNA binding, increased LE cells, low C3 and C4) together with proteinuria, and nephrotic syndrome with or without renal failure.

Treatment
There are limited clinical trials available and most clinicians concur that careful follow-up of individual patients is mandatory. Patients with minimal, focal and membranous lesions

have a good prognosis and do not require treatment with steroids or other immunosuppressive therapy, unless required for symptomatic arthritis or other multisystem manifestation of the disease. Patients with proliferative lesions who usually have heavy proteinuria or nephrotic syndrome require steroids, initially in high doses (1−2 mg/kg of prednisolone per day), reducing the dosage preferably to an alternate-day regimen for long-term maintenance. Some physicians add azathioprine (or rarely cyclophosphamide) as a 'steroid sparing' adjunct to therapy or to patients who respond poorly to steroids alone. Long-term treatment is monitored by the clinical state of the patient, renal function, proteinuria, ESR, anti-DNA titre, complement levels and immune complexes. However, most physicians treating large groups of patients with SLE rely more on clinical assessment than serological testing. Occasionally, patients suffer with acute exacerbation of the disease when pulse therapy with methylprednisolone (1.0 g i.v. over 15 minutes daily for 2−3 days), or even plasmaphoresis, has been tried.

Dialysis and transplantation in patients with SLE
Limited experience has shown that patients with SLE do well on haemodialysis. In many patients, the disease appears to 'burn out' and steroids may be reduced or stopped. There may be a risk of developing other non-renal organ problems, e.g. myocarditis, hepatitis or cerebral problems. Therefore, clinical and serological monitoring of the patient is essential.

There is no contraindication to transplantation since the disease rarely recurs in a transplant graft. One particular problem is that many patients with SLE have white blood cell antibodies, thus limiting the choice of kidneys available.

Vasculitis

Vasculitis occurs in a variety of conditions, including Henoch−Schönlein purpura and SLE, but discussion here is limited to two conditions: polyarteritis and Wegener's granulomatosis, where the kidneys are likely to be involved. Men are more commonly affected than women.

Polyarteritis
This is classically divided into the microscopic variety and polyarteritis nodosa.

Microscopic polyarteritis presents with fevers, skin rashes, abdominal pain, asthma, neuropathy and renal involvement (proteinuria, haematuria, nephrotic syndrome, rarely renal failure — rapidly progressive disease) and hypertension (occasionally malignant). Eosinophilia, a raised ESR, cryoglobulinaemia and circulating immune complexes, may be found. Hepatitis B antigen is present in some patients. Renal failure may develop or progress. Renal biopsy shows a proliferative glomerulonephritis with areas of necrosis. Immunoflourescence reveals little staining with either immunoglobulins or complement, but fibrin may be present. Vessels show minor inflammatory changes only, with occasional deposits of IgM and C3. Antineutrophil cytoplasmic antibodies may be positive.

Polyarteritis nodosa (macroscopic polyarteritis) affects larger vessels (> 100 μm diameter). Hypertension is a predominant feature. Lung involvement is less common. Hepatitis B antigen may be present. Angiography of visceral vessels may show microaneurysms, especially in the kidney and in the territory of the coeliac artery. Renal failure develops in untreated patients although not as rapidly as with the microscopic variety.

Treatment of both types is with steroids initially, using prednisolone 1 mg/kg per day tapering slowly as the disease comes under control, together with cyclophosphamide 2 mg/kg. Plasmaphoeresis has been used in patients requiring dialysis. Azathioprine is usually substituted for cyclophamide long-term.

Wegener's granulomatosis
This is an arteritic and granulomatous condition affecting the face and upper and lower respiratory tract, with occasional vasculitic lesions elsewhere, including the kidney. Mild renal failure, with proteinuria and haematuria is common and, if untreated, progresses rapidly to a crescentic nephritis. Treatment with steroids and cyclophosphamide is effective with

plasma exchange being used for severe cases. Antineutrophil cytoplasmic antibodies may be positive.

In contrast to SLE, patients with vasculitis may present a problem when on dialysis. The disease tends to be progressive, making vascular access difficult. Gangrene of limbs may occur. Risks of transplantation have not been fully assessed.

The kidney and bacterial endocarditis

Unexplained proteinuria and haematuria with features of glomerulonephritis on biopsy in a patient with a heart murmur, should alert the physician to the possibility of bacterial endocarditis. Renal biopsy appearances vary from focal and segmental changes in subacute cases to proliferative changes in acute endocarditis. There are widespread deposits of immunoglobulins and complement showing that the lesion is an immune complex nephritis. The lesion heals when the endocarditis is treated.

6.6 Non-arteritic 'vascular' lesions affecting the kidney

There are a group of conditions which have in common non-arteritic vascular damage associated with a histological change termed 'fibrinoid necrosis'. Although the origin of the change is unclear, patients with this abnormality sometimes share abnormalities of the coagulation system and evidence of haemolysis. The conditions showing these changes include scleroderma, haemolytic uraemic syndrome, malignant hypertension (p. 185), post-partum acute renal failure (p. 95), transplant rejection, radiation nephritis (p. 160), as well as SLE and polyarteritis nodosa (p. 93).

Scleroderma

This is, fortunately, a rare cause of renal failure with a bad prognosis. Renal failure develops rapidly, often with evidence of haemolysis. Hypertension may or may not be present. It has been suggested that the angiotensin-converting enzyme-inhibitor, captopril is useful in preventing rapid acceleration of renal disease but this has not been our experience. Patients with scleroderma have multiple problems on haemodialysis. Therefore, either peritoneal dialysis or transplantation would appear to be the optimum policy for these unfortunate people.

Haemolytic uraemic syndrome

Haemolytic uraemic syndrome occurs mainly in children and a similar condition, *thrombotic thrombocytopenic purpura*, occurs in adults. Renal involvement is more common in children, and widespread lesions, in adults. In both, the disease may be preceded by a bacterial or viral infection — in children, by gastro-enteritis due to a verucotoxin producing *E. coli*. The widespread clinical effects (bleeding, jaundice, neurological disorders, including disturbed levels of consciousness and fits) presumably reflect widespread ischaemic damage due to intravascular thrombosis. Investigation reveals a haemolytic anaemia with abnormal red cell forms, thrombocytopenia, raised fibrin degradation products, lowered fibrinogen levels, raised bilirubin and renal failure.

Treatment
Despite claims to the contrary, heparin has not been shown to be effective in any controlled trial. Most cases in children recover spontaneously even after one or two haemodialyses. Plasma exchange or plasma infusion (to restore clotting factors) is claimed to be beneficial. In adults, steroids, antiplatelet drugs and prostacyclin have also been given in uncontrolled trials.

Post-partum acute renal failure

This is a rare complication of pregnancy occurring 2−3 weeks after delivery. There is usually a preceding febrile illness immediately post-partum, followed 2 weeks later by oliguria, hypertension renal failure, evidence of disseminated intravascular coagulation, and haemolysis. Treatment with heparin has been claimed to be successful but has to be given early.

Most patients have developed irreversible renal failure with severe intractable hypertension which may only respond to bilateral nephrectomy.

6.7 The kidney in diabetes mellitus and rheumatoid arthritis (RA)

Diabetes mellitus

Urinary tract infections are said to be more common in patients with diabetes but the evidence is inconclusive. Certain organisms, e.g. coagulase positive staphylococci, occur more frequently and, if associated with acute pyelonephritis, may result in acute papillary necrosis.

Diabetic glomerulosclerosis
This condition is usually associated with other diabetic microangiopathies, including retinopathy and neuropathy. Insulin-dependent diabetics are at a special risk, and present with proteinuria, nephrotic syndrome or renal failure. Biopsy, preferably with ultrasound, shows increase of the mesangial matrix (diabetic glomerulosclerosis) and widening of the capillary basement membranes. 'Nodular' lesions occur in about 20% of cases. Pyelography is best avoided in patients with diabetes, since irreversible renal failure may be precipitated.

Microalbuminuria
Normal urine contains minute quantities of albumin (<15 µg per minute). It has been shown that an albumin secretion rate above 15 µg per minute ('Microalbuminuria'), is associated with the likely development of diabetic glomerulosclerosis; for which there is no specific treatment. It is, however, hoped that better control of diabetes and any associated hypertension (using angiotension converting enzyme inhibitors or calcium channel blocking drugs rather than β-blockers) may reduce the incidence of diabetic glomerulosclerosis and associated complications, including retinopathy and vascular disease.

Rheumatoid arthritis

The development of proteinuria or renal failure in a patient with rheumatoid arthritis may be due to:
- amyloidosis
- membranous nephritis if the patient is taking gold or penicillamine
- papillary necrosis in those with a history of analgesic abuse.

6.8 Amyloidosis and paraproteinaemia

Renal amyloid may occur with a variety of predisposing disorders (Table 6.5).

Amyloidosis is closely associated with *paraproteinuria*. This is a generic term which includes a number of different entities:
- multiple myeloma
- Waldenström's macroglobulinaemia
- mixed cryoglobulinaemias

Details of these conditions are given in Table 6.6.

6.9 Histology of various renal lesions

See Figures 6.4–6.25 (see pp. 99–108).

Table 6.5 Predisposing disorders of renal amyloid.

Predisposing disorder	Precursor protein
Immunocyte dyscrasia (myeloma, light chain disease)	AL fibrils from light chains
Chronic active disease (infections, rheumatoid arthritis)	AA fibrils from serum amyloid A protein
Familial Mediterranean fever	AA fibrils from serum amyloid A protein
Long-term haemodialysis (amyloid mainly localized in periarticular tissue and bone)	β_2-microglobulin

Table 6.6 Forms of paraproteinaemia.

Disease	Renal presentation	Biochemistry	Histology		Treatment
			Glomeruli	Tubules interstitium	
Multiple myeloma including kappa and lambda light chains nephropathics	Proteinuria, acute renal failure, chronic renal failure, hypercalcaemia, hyperuricaemia, renal vein thrombosin	Paraprotein band, Bence–Jones protein, selective $\uparrow$ in immunoglobulin	Amyloid	Giant cells, casts, interstitial infiltration	Melphalan and other cytotoxic regimens, plasma exchange for acute failure associated with light chains
Macroglobulinaemia	Hyperviscosity with renal failure (rare)	Plasma viscosity $\uparrow$, IgM $\uparrow\uparrow$	Amyloid, capillary thrombi with deposits containing IgM	Casts	Plasma exchange, cytotoxic agents
Mixed cryoglobulinaemia	Acute nephritic syndrome, acute renal failure, secondary to other renal lesions (?)	Cryoglobulins	Proliferative glomerulonephritis, capillary thrombi	Variable interstitial infiltrate with vasculitic changes	Plasma exchange, steroids cytotoxic agents (for acute exacerbations)

$\uparrow$: increase; $\uparrow\uparrow$: marked increase

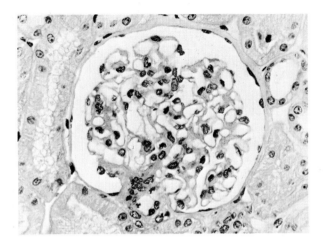

Fig. 6.4 Minimal change GN: light microscopy showing normal glomerulus.

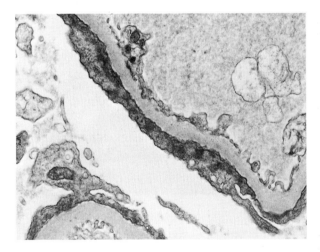

Fig. 6.5 Minimal change GN: electron microscopy showing foot process fusion.

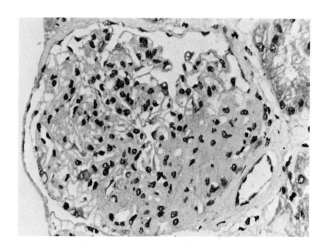

Fig. 6.6 Focal glomerulosclerosis: light microscopy.

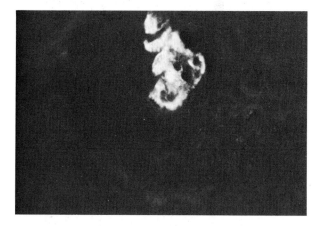

Fig. 6.7 Focal glomerulosclerosis: immunofluorescence showing IgM trapped in sclerosed area of glomerulus.

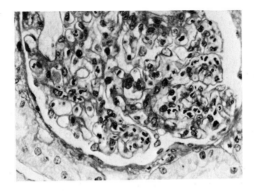

Fig. 6.8 Acute proliferative (post-streptococcal) GN: light microscopy.

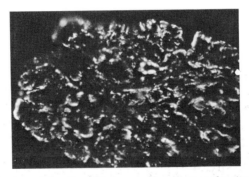

Fig. 6.9 Acute proliferative GN: immunofluorescence showing IgG in granular deposits along capillary wall

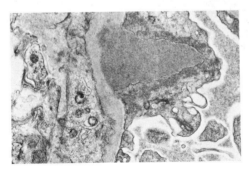

Fig. 6.10 Acute proliferative GN: electron microscopy showing electron dense 'hump' on outer (epithelial) aspect of capillary basement membrane.

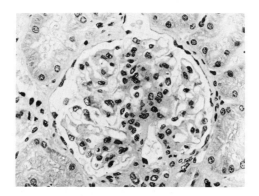

Fig. 6.11 Focal and segmental GN: light microscopy showing focal mesangial cell proliferation.

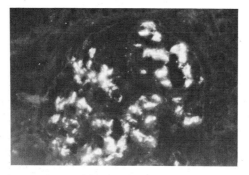

Fig. 6.12 Focal and segmental GN: immunofluorescence showing widespread deposits of mesangial IgA

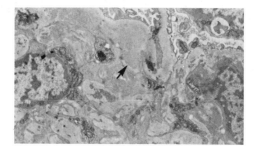

Fig. 6.13 Focal and segmental GN: electron microscopy showing mesangial electron dense deposits (arrowed).

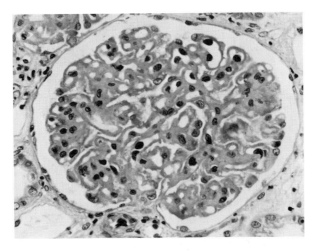

Fig. 6.14 Membranous GN: light microscopy.

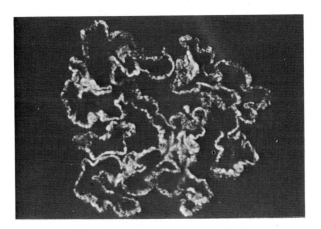

Fig. 6.15 Membranous GN: immunofluorescence showing discrete granular deposits of IgG along capillary wall.

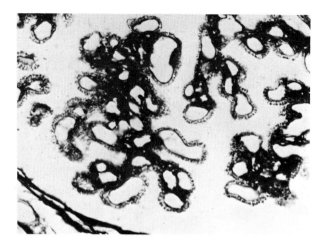

Fig. 6.16 Membranous GN: light microscopy with silver (basement membrane) stain showing projections ('spiking') on epithelial side of basement membrane.

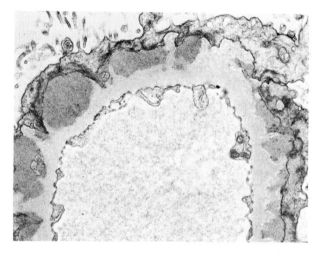

Fig. 6.17 Membranous GN: electron microscopy showing discrete electron dense deposits along outer (epithelial) border of basement membrane.

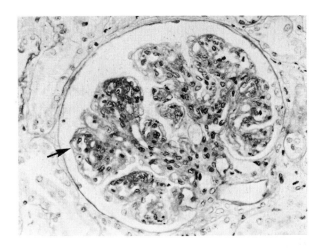

Fig. 6.18 Mesangio-capillary GN: light microscopy showing proliferative changes which highlight the 'lobular' pattern. Note the double contour of the basement membrane ('tram-lining') (arrowed).

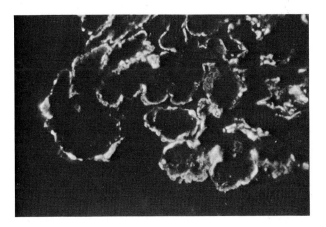

Fig. 6.19 Mesangio-capillary GN: immunofluorescence staining with IgG.

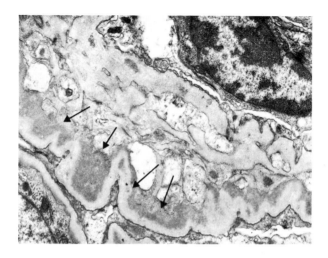

Fig. 6.20 Mesangio-capillary GN: electron microscopy showing subendothelial deposits (arrowed).

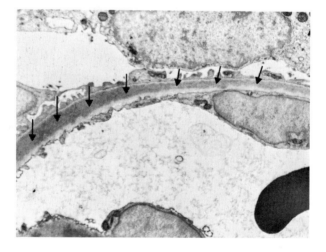

Fig. 6.21 Mesangio-capillary GN: electron microscopy showing dense deposits within capillary basement membrane (arrowed).

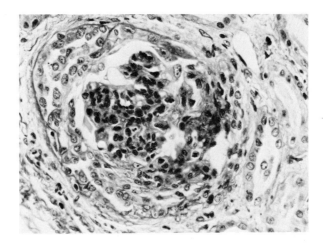

Fig. 6.22 Rapidly progressive GN: light microscopy showing crescent.

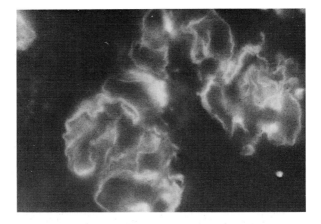

Fig. 6.23 Rapidly progressive glomerulonephritis: immunoflourescence showing anti glomerulerbasement membrane antibody deposited in 'linear' fashion along capillary basement membrane. (Courtesy of Professor D.J. Evans).

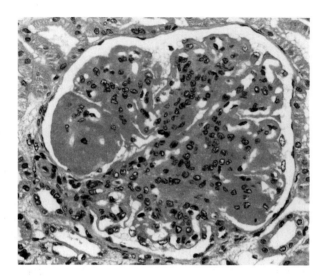

Fig. 6.24 Diabetes showing diabeteic glomerulosclerosis.

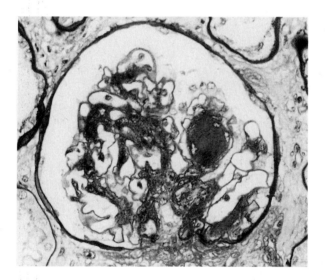

Fig. 6.25 Haemolytic uraemic syndrome showing increased mesangial matrix and capillary thrombi.

7: Dialysis and transplantation

7.1 Introduction

The three forms of treatment for patients with end-stage renal failure should be regarded as complimentary and available in any one centre. All three methods have improved over the past 20 years. Haemodialysis has become easier with modern automated proportionators and disposable dialysers. Continuous ambulatory peritoneal dialysis (CAPD) has largely replaced intermittent peritoneal dialysis. Blood transfusion, improved immunosuppressive drugs and better matching between donor and recipient have improved graft survival. Indications and contraindications to the three forms of treatment are given in Table 7.1.

Table 7.1 Indications and contraindications to end-stage renal failure.

	Haemodialysis	CAPD	Transplantation
Relative indication	Age < 60 years	Age > 60 years Diabetes	Age < 40 years Diabetes
Relative contraindication	Scleroderma Diabetes	Extensive abdominal surgery	Age > 60 years, bladder surgery
	Cardiovascular instability		

The choice for any renal unit is governed by available resources. Most units would not dialyse or transplant patients with severe mental disorders, malignancy, amputations or severe cerebrovascular disease.

Timing of dialysis and transplantation

Haemo- or peritoneal dialysis should start before the more serious complications of uraemia (bleeding tendency, clinical neuropathy, pericarditis) occur, or when the GFR reaches about 4 ml per minute with a corresponding plasma creatinine concentration of 1000–1200 μmol/l, depending on the patient's size. On balance, it is better to start haemo- or peritoneal dialysis before transplantation (to improve the metabolic consequences of chronic renal failure), although successful transplantation has been undertaken without prior dialysis.

7.2 Haemodialysis methods

Blood access

Ideally, a fistula should have been made at least 6 weeks before starting dialysis. If this has not been possible, either a Scribner (A–V) shunt is inserted into a leg leaving arms free for fistulae later, or a internal jugular catheter is inserted until the fistula is usable.

Blood access
- subclavian or internal jugular catheters
- AV fistulae
- Scribner shunts
- other vascular access

Subclavian or internal jugular catheters are being increasingly used for temporary or permanent vascular access. Great care is required for their insertion. Single or double lumen temporary catheters are available; a permanent catheter (Francis or Perm-cath) is available and has to be inserted by a surgical procedure. Temporary catheters may be and permanent catheters are always tunnelled to reduce the risk of infection. All patients with catheters have a check chest X-ray prior to dialysis.

Complications of subclavian and internal jugular catheters include: thrombosis of catheter lumens; infection; subclavian vein stenosis leading to swollen arms and subsequent problems in establishing AV fistulae — this is less likely with internal jugular vein catheters.

AV fistulae
AV fistulae are usually fashioned from the radial artery to the cephalic vein but other anastomoses may be used e.g. ulnar artery to ulnar vein or brachial artery to brachial vein.

Care of fistulae
Fistulae rarely clot or become infected, and have a life of several years. Occasionally stenoses, which require further vascular surgery, occur.

Scribner shunts
The original Scribner shunt is still in widespread use. Preferred sites of insertion include radial artery to cephalic vein or post tibial artery to long saphenous vein in the leg. The venous limb lasts on average 6−8 months and the arterial limb 2−3 years and various complications can occur.
1 Clotting, which occurs when signs of malfunction (poor arterial flow, high venous pressure) are present and may be prevented by early resiting, anticoagulants and avoidance of kinking, hypotension and cold. Repeated clotting episodes usually indicate the need for shunt revision. A 'shuntogram' is helpful to outline the arterial and venous circulations.
2 Infection — avoided by strict aseptic technique.
3 Disconnection — avoided by careful patient and nursing education.

Several varieties of shunts are available (including the original 'Scribner' shunt), e.g. Thomas shunt (for femoral access) or Busselmeir shunt, although these less conventional ones have been replaced by fistulae and grafts.

Other vascular access
Various alternatives to shunts and fistulae have been described, including Dacron prostheses, bovine arteries and autologous vein grafts. These have been placed in thighs, lower and upper-arm sites. Most recently, an implant using biocarbon has been described which does not require needling. Doubtless, further improvement in vascular access will continue to occur.

Dialysis hardware

Water supply
Softened mains water has been used extensively as the sole water purification. Within the last few years, however, renal units in areas where mains water contains aluminium in excess of 50 µmol/l (possibly in excess of 20 µmol/l) have treated water with reversed osmosis.

Proportionators
Most renal units have single-pass proportionating systems which prepare fluid from a 'concentrate' mixed with treated water to form dialysate of physiological composition. A typical formula (mmol/l) is Na^+ 140, K^+ 1.5, Ca^{2+} 1.5, Mg^{2+} 0.5, Cl^- 100, acetate 35, Dextrose 12. The dialysate is deaerated, warmed to 37°C and monitored for conductivity (sodium concentration) before going to the dialyser. Dialysis fluid returns from the dialyser to be checked for blood leaks, and passes through an effluent pump before going to a drain. A number of fail-safe alarms and controls are required to monitor conductivity, negative ('dialysate') pressure, venous pressure, venous bubble-trap blood level, arterial cushion pressure, mains water pressure and mains electricity supply. Proportionating machines have improved in design, and are becoming less bulky due to improved electronics. Most have built-in blood pumps, heparin pumps and facilities to change from haemodialysis to ultrafiltration; most vary the sodium content of the dialysate and have easy adaptation for either acetate or bicarbonate dialysis. For a dialysis circuit, see Fig. 7.1.

Dialysis and dialysers
The physical laws governing dialysis include diffusion, ultrafiltration and convection. The original dialysis membrane used was cuprophane but other more porous membranes (polycarbonate, polysulphone and polyacrilonitrile (PAN) membranes) have been increasingly used allowing clearances of substances of a higher molecular weight. Typical clearances of cuprophane and polysulphone membranes are shown in Table 7.2.

There are now a bewildering number of disposable dialysers

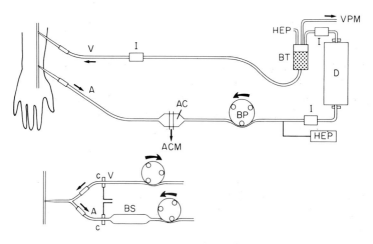

Fig. 7.1 A diagram of a dialysis circuit. The upper diagram shows conventional two needle dialysis. The lower diagram shows 'single needle' dialysis where one or two blood pumps may be used with clamps (C) on the arterial and venous line. If two blood pumps are used a blood sac (BS) is utilized in the circuit. V: venous line; A: arterial line; I: infusion points. BT: bubble trap; HEP: alternative sites for heparin infusion; VPM: venous pressure monitor. D: dialyser; BP: blood pump; AC: arterial cushion; and ACM: arterial cushion monitor.

Table 7.2 Clearances of cuprophane and polysulphone membranes (ml/min).

Substance	Molecular weight	Cuprophane clearance	Polysulphone clearance
Urea	60	150	189
Creatinine	113	100	168
Uric acid	165	100	NA
EDTA	380	65	NA
B_{12}	1355	40	118
Inulin	5175	20	86
β_2 microglobulin	12000	NIL	56

NB Ultrafiltration through a high flux polysulphone membrane is very high and has to be controlled by a volumetric pump system in the proportionating machine. (NA = not available.)

which utilize different membranes of various thickness, flat-plate and hollow-fibre designs, different geometric construction and variable surface areas. All have low residual blood volumes. The ideal dialyser should have a wide range of clearances, including β_2-microglobulin (molecular weight 12 000), adequate ultrafiltration, low residual blood volume, and be reasonably priced. Many would add that dialysers should be capable of reuse several times without loss of efficiency. Monitoring of new dialysers takes place regularly in the UK at the University of Newcastle on Tyne, by Dr N.A. Hoenich, and the results are published regularly by the Department of Health (see Appendix 9).

Haemodialysis and haemofiltration

Haemodialysis is the form of treatment conventionally practised and usually involves simultaneous diffusion and ultrafiltration. Some patients tolerate simultaneous diffusion and ultrafiltration poorly and may undergo sequential diffusion and ultrafiltration during which the blood pressure is maintained by keeping a constant osmolality and peripheral resistance. Since there is no significant solute loss during ultrafiltration the total hours of treatment have to be increased.

Haemofiltration is an extension of ultrafiltration during which 20–30 litres of ultrafiltrate is removed through a very porous membrane and replaced by some physiological equivalent. Special fluid controlled monitoring systems are required for this form of dialysis which has been claimed to give superior control of blood pressure, less anaemia, bone disease, improved blood lipids and less side-effects during treatment. Haemofiltration is 2–3 times as expensive as haemodialysis. *High flux dialysers* are being used to increase dialysis clearances of large molecular weight substances but also require fluid control monitoring systems.

Haemodiafiltration is a compromise of these techniques when a simultaneous dialysis and smaller amounts (4–6 litres) of ultrafiltration is undertaken.

Plasmaphoresis can now be undertaken using plasma filters in a dialysis circuit with careful ultrafiltration control.

Dialysis techniques

There are a great variety of dialysis needles and lines. Most units now use disposable dialysers, some reusing dialysers between one and five times. A diagram of a dialysis circuit is given in Figure 7.1.

There is considerable debate about the assessment of the adequacy of dialysis. In general, dialysis hours have been reduced as dialyser efficiency has improved. An analysis of the United States Cooperative study by Gotch and Sargent (*Kidney International* **28**; 526−534: 1985) suggested that adequate dialysis is achieved if Kt/V is > 1.0, where K is dialyser urea clearance, t is treatment time, V is body urea distribution volume.

Ideally Kt/V should be calculated by computer but several easier mathematical equations are under assessment. It should be stressed that there is a need for a sufficient protein intake to maintain a protein catabolic rate of 1.2. High flux dialysers have allowed a reduction in dialysis hours to 6−12 per week tailored to the patient's individual requirements. Whatever the schedule, periodic checks of the patient's clinical condition are mandatory and should include the following.

1 Full clinical examination including weight, blood pressure, 'squatting test' (for proximal myopathy), examination of the abdomen, fundi, and central nervous system, including ankle jerks and vibration sense in feet.

2 Full blood count, urea, electrolytes, creatinine, calcium, phosphate, alkaline phosphatase levels, liver function tests, hepatitis B antigen, hepatitis C antibody, ferritin, β_2 microglobulin, parathyroid hormone.

3 Chest X-ray 6−12 monthly; skeletal survey every 12 months.

Diet

The use of high-efficiency dialysers has resulted in a more liberal protein allowance of about 80−100 g protein per day. Patients should be warned about high potassium and high phosphate foods (see Appendix 6). At one time a high-calorie intake was encouraged (especially with fats) but the wisdom of this has been challenged in view of the incidence of atheroma in a dialysis population.

Drugs

Patients on dialysis are usually routinely given a multi-vitamin (Orovite or equivalent) and combination iron and folic acid tablet (e.g. Folex 350). In addition, a number of other tablets will inevitably be given for a variety of complications.

Physiological consequences of haemodialysis

Representative changes in the composition of the blood in patients on haemodialysis are given in the Table 7.3.

A number of consequences result from changes during dialysis. They may be summarized as follows.

1 Although the blood pH and bicarbonate rises as bicarbonate is generated from acetate, cerebrospinal fluid (CSF) pH and bicarbonate lags behind. However, CSF P_{CO_2} rises in association with reduced ventilation. This lag effect may be responsible for 'disequilibrium', headaches, restlessness, disorientation, or fits (seen more commonly in acute renal failure).

2 The fall in P_{O_2} is probably due to pulmonary microemboli activated by the alternative pathway of complement. This is associated with a sharp fall in the white blood cell count. The fall in P_{O_2} combined with anaemia reduces tissue oxygen release by up to 15%, which negates the advantage gained by the increase in 2-3 diphosphoglycerate found during alkalosis. The combined hypoxia and reduced oxygen delivery may be exacerbated in patients with cardiorespiratory problems and oxygen may be needed during dialysis. These changes in P_{O_2} are not seen if bicarbonate dialysate is used, and are less using non-cuprophane membranes.

3 The increased sodium concentration may lead to thirst with excess water intake in the post-dialysis period.

4 The fall in potassium is governed by the dialysate potassium concentration and surface area of the dialyser. Precipitate

Table 7.3 Changes in the composition of blood.

	Pre-dialysis	At end of dialysis	
		Blood	CSF
pH	7.3	7.5	7.3
P_{CO_2} (mmHg)	35	35	35
P_{O_2} (mmHg)	80	65	
HCO_3^- (mmol/l)	15	25	15
Na^+ (mmol/l)	136	144	
K^+ (mmol/l)	6.0	3.0	
Urea (mmol/l)	39	5.0	
Creatinine (μmol/l)	1200	400	
Ca^{2+} (mmol/l)	2.4	2.9	
PO_4^{3-} (mmol/l)	2.5	1.5	
Osmolality (mmol/kg)	325	300	

falls in potassium may be associated with arrhythmias in patients with heart disease and confusion in patients with co-existent liver disease.

5 The urea and creatinine differences give some clue to the efficiency of dialysis. Persistently high (or low) urea levels with average predialysis creatinine levels suggest over- (or under-) protein intake. Some muscular patients have high levels of creatinine.

6 Since the bath calcium is ionized the total serum calcium tends to rise slightly but rarely above 3 mmol/l post-dialysis.

7 The reduction in serum phosphate is not matched by a reduction in intracellular red cell phosphate.

8 The reduction in osmolality may play a part in the development of symptomatic hypotension (see below).

9 Bicarbonate is generated from acetate through the Krebs cycle. Acetate intolerance is thought by some to induce headaches, vomiting, hypotension and post-dialysis inertia. Bicarbonate dialysate is being increasingly used in many haemodialysis centres.

7.3 Complications during dialysis

Hypotension

Nearly all patients suffer, at some time, episodes of hypotension during dialysis, associated with vomiting, diarrhoea, fainting and, occasionally, arrhythmias and angina. This usually occurs if high ultrafiltration is required due to excess weight gain between dialyses. Various remedies have been tried to counter hypotension, including:

- reassessing the patient's 'dry' weight and adjusting dialysis accordingly
- continued admonition to the patient to prevent unnecessary weight gains
- increasing dialysis hours using smaller dialysers with less ultrafiltration
- increasing dialysis frequency from 2 to 3 times a week
- increasing conductivity (sodium concentration) from 140 to 144 mmol/l
- use of Slow sodium tablets (10 mmol/tablet) before and during dialysis
- giving $100-200$ ml of 2 N saline during dialysis
- use of ACE inhibitors (e.g. enalapril $5-10$ mg daily) to inhibit thirst
- changing from an acetate to a bicarbonate dialysis

Headaches and vomiting

Between 30–50% of all dialysis patients are affected, although often without significant changes in blood pressure. The aetiology is uncertain but the migraine-like nature of such complications would suggest a vascular basis. Several remedies have been tried, including:

- anti-nausea preparation, e.g. prochlorperazine (25 mg pre-dialysis)
- metoclopramide 10 mg, or Paramax, 1–2 tablets, pre-dialysis
- diazepam 5 mg pre- or during dialysis
- propranolol 10 mg or clonidine 25 µg pre-dialysis
- changing from acetate to bicarbonate dialysis

Technical complications

(see Fig. 7.1)

High venous pressure
The venous line should be checked for kinks and the blood flow measured. Negative pressure should be reduced, and if blood flow is poor, the dialyser line should be warmed. Venous spasms can occur with cold saline or after drugs given i.v. Persistently high venous pressure indicates malfunctioning of shunt or fistula which may need resiting.

Low venous pressure
This occasionally occurs if the patient is positioned lower than the dialyser, but is usually due to low blood pressure, kinked lines or a poorly positioned arterial needle. *It is important to set the venous pressure alarm close to the indicating needle as a low venous pressure may be the only indication of some serious mishap, e.g. disconnection of blood lines.*

Blood leaks
Leaks rarely occur with the more widespread use of disposable dialysers.

Blood flows
Optimum blood flows are 250–300 ml per minute, or higher if shorter dialysis schedules are used. Below 200 ml per minute dialysis becomes inefficient. Poor blood flows are usually due to poor shunt or fistula function, occasionally to hypotension.

Disconnection of line
Disconnection may result in massive blood loss or air embolism and is therefore the most serious of all technical complications. Fortunately, it is extremely rare and is largely preventable by: (a) correct 'bridging' of all blood lines; and (b) correct adjustment of all machine alarms.

Clotted blood lines
These are due either to poor blood flows with cooling of lines, or insufficient heparin administration. The usual dose of heparin given to adults is 5000 u pre-dialysis with 1500–2000 u per hour during dialysis. Whole blood clotting times are usually undertaken in the first few dialyses to establish heparin dosage.

Blood recirculation
Recirculation of blood around the dialyser occurs if fistula needles are inserted too close together. This is an occasional cause of 'underdialysis' and is spotted by simultaneously taking blood for urea and creatinine concentration tests from the arterial line compared to an opposite arm vein. Normally, these values should be the same but recirculation results in lower arterial line urea and creatinine concentration levels, compared to blood elsewhere in the circulation.

Febrile reactions
'Rigors' may be due either to sepsis or pyrogenic reactions associated with dialyser reuse. Fevers on dialysis require a careful search for any likely cause and should include careful clinical examination and blood cultures.

Hard-water reactions
Reaction against hard water produces nausea, vomiting and

headache 4−6 hours after dialysis commences. Water should be tested for hardness prior to every dialysis; frequent regeneration of water softeners is required.

Power or water pressure failure
Such failures activate a battery-operated mains alarm. Patients should be instructed to use a manual pump to rinse back blood lines and come off dialysis.

Complications occurring between dialyses

Clotted shunts and fistulae
Although it is important to declot shunts and fistulae promptly, an attempt should be made to determine the cause of the clotting, e.g. low blood pressure, tight clothing, insufficient anticoagulation. Some patients may clot shunts repeatedly, and anticoagulation with warfarin, or the use of antiplatelet drugs such as sulphinpyrazone (100 mg b.d.), or low dose aspirin (75 mg) may be tried.

Infected shunts and fistulae
Any infection in a dialysis patient requires prompt bacteriological investigation and treatment. Shunt infections are usually caused by *Staphylococcus aureus*; rarely, by other Gram-positive or negative infections. Treatment should begin after bacteriological samples have been taken since septicaemia is common. A suitable combination of antimicrobial agents includes flucloxacillin (250 mg q.d.s.). cephalexin (500 mg o.d.), tobramycin (1 mg/kg at the end of dialysis) or vancomycin (1.0 g in 250 ml N saline) over 2 hours, every 10 days, and covers most shunt infections.

7.4 Long-term problems of patients on haemodialysis

Patients on maintenance haemodialysis are subject to a variety of long-term complications.

Renal bone disease

Calcium and phosphate metabolism has already been discussed in Chapter 5.

Hyperparathyroidism
Most patients on haemodialysis have a raised parathormone level, fewer have radiological changes, and fewer still, symptoms. Measures to prevent the development of hyperparathyroidism include the following.
1 A dialysis solution calcium content of 1.5 mmol/l.
2 Control of phosphate intake and absorption by dietary restriction aluminium hydroxide. Aluminium should only be given for short periods (6 weeks maximum). Persistent hyperphosphataemia thereafter may be treated with either calcium carbonate (e.g. Calcichew 1 b.d. or t.d.s.) and lowering the dialysate calcium to 1.0 or 0.75 mmol/l, or oral magnesium carbonate (0.5–1.5 g/day) with withdrawal of dialysate magnesium. Newer calcium salts (e.g. calcium acetate) and vitamin D metabolites (e.g. 22 oxacalcitriol) are awaited with interest.
3 The administration of vitamin D_3, preferably as the renal metabolite 1-25 $(OH)_2D_3$ (calcitriol), starting at a dose of 0.25 μg once or twice a day. It would seem preferable to give calcitriol early in the course of dialysis to prevent radiological changes rather than treat changes once they occur. Careful monitoring of dosage is required in order to prevent hypercalcaemia or hyperphosphataemia.
4 i.v. calcitriol or alfacalcidol is under review.
5 Some patients develop worsening hyperparathyroidism despite prophylaxis or treatment with calcitriol, and should then undergo a total parathyroidectomy.

Osteomalacia
Osteomalacia results in a proximal myopathy and fractures, and may progress to a crippling bone disease. It is now recognized that there are two types.
1 That associated with vitamin D deficiency and responding to cholecalciferol (0.05–1.0 mg per day) or 1-25 $(OH)_2D_3$

(calcitrol) (0.5−1.0 μg per day). This variety of osteomalacia may follow a parathyroidectomy.

2 That which does not respond to vitamin D_3 and due to aluminium intoxication, which also includes dialysis dementia (p. 125).

Histologically, the appearances or both types of osteomalacia are similar. The diagnosis requires measurement of mains water and plasma aluminium levels, and by bone biopsy.

Cardiovascular complications

Hypertension
(see Chapter 11)
Patients may be divided into three groups.
1 Those with 'volume-dependent' hypertension whose blood pressure comes under control with weight removal.
2 Those with 'renin-dependent' hypertension whose blood pressure is often worsened by weight removal and who need hypotensive drugs (e.g. atenalol, nifedipine or captopril).
3 Those with normal blood pressure who may become hypotensive on dialysis, requiring sodium supplements.

In practice, many patients find it difficult to achieve volume depletion sufficient to normalize blood pressure. They experience cramps and hypotension on dialysis and thirst and general malaise between dialyses. Some of these patients need hypotensive therapy which is best avoided on the day of dialysis.

Atherosclerosis
The combination of long-standing hypertension and abnormal blood lipids results in accelerated atherosclerosis, with myocardial infarction a likely consequence. The use of lipid-lowering agents is under review.

Pericarditis
Pericarditis occurs infrequently in a dialysis population. Most attacks are associated with a haemopericardium; rarely with tamponade. Any patient with unexplained hypotension should be carefully investigated with echocardiography, to exclude a pericardial effusion. Treatment consists of changing to short,

frequent dialyses with minimum heparin and the use of indomethacin 25 mg t.d.s. Most attacks resolve spontaneously without pericardial aspiration or operation.

Pulmonary oedema
Most attacks of pulmonary oedema in dialysis patients are due to salt and water overload and ultrafiltration will return the heart size to normal. In a few older, male, patients, continuous overload (with excessive weight gain between dialysis) results in a form of congestive cardiomyopathy with gross cardio-megaly, hypotension and a poor cardiac output. The prognosis is poor. In some of these patients, admission to hospital for frequent haemodialysis, careful control of fluid intake, use of digoxin and/or a vasodilator drug (e.g. isosorbide) occasionally helps.

Hepatic complications

Patients on dialysis are subject to attacks of viral hepatitis. The majority of these attacks are hepatitis B antigen negative and, as hepatitis A antibody titres do not change, it is likely that the attack is due to hepatitis C virus. Most attacks are asymptomatic and revealed only by a rise in transaminases. Other causes of 'transaminitis' include cytomegalovirus infec-tion, toxoplasmosis, Epstein–Barr virus and iron overload. Most attacks are self-limiting and require only observation and avoidance of hepatotoxic drugs, or drugs metabolized by the liver (e.g. warfarin).

Hepatitis B infections have occurred in dialysis units and occasionally patients who are hepatitis B-positive will need dialysis. Passive immunization with hepatitis B-antisera is available for staff inadvertently exposed to hepatitis B-infec-tion. Active immunization against hepatitis B is also available and should be offered to all staff working in renal units.

Chronic liver disease occurs infrequently among a dialysis population. A variety of abnormal histology is found in these patients, including chronic active hepatitis with piecemeal necrosis leading to cirrhosis, 'lobular' hepatitis, iron overload, refractile bodies (silicone from dialysis lines?) and mild non-specific inflammation in the portal tracts. High ferritin levels should be avoided by limiting parenteral iron therapy and monitoring ferritin levels.

Renal complications

Renal complications include acquired renal cystic disease and the development of malignancies within cysts.

Neurological complications

- peripheral neuropathy is only seen in inadequately dialysed patients
- restless legs' (a form of neuropathy?) is an unpleasant nocturnal complication which may be helped by 0.5−1.0 mg clonazepam
- subarachnoid haemorrhage occurs in patients with polycystic kidneys who have an increased incidence of berry aneurysm compared to patients with other forms of renal disease
- Subdural haematomas (spontaneous or traumatic) have been described in patients on dialysis. Any patient with unexplained headaches of focal neurological signs should have a CT brain scan.

Aluminium intoxication

Aluminium intoxication among dialysis patients may lead to:
- hypochromic anaemia
- bone disease (see p. 122)
- dialysis dementia

Aluminium intoxication may be avoided by using dialysis fluid with a low aluminium content (should be less than 50 μmol/l) and avoidance of aluminium hydroxide for phosphate binding. Serum aluminium levels should be monitored.
- aluminium level < 0.7 μmol/l (20 μg/l) − normal

- aluminium level 0.7−3.7 μmol/l (20−100 μg/l) − no toxicity
- aluminium level 3.7−7.7 μmol/l (100−200 μg/l) − at risk of toxicity
- aluminium level >7.4 μmol/l (>200 μg/l) − toxicity to be expected.

Aluminium toxicity has also been assessed by using the desferrioxamine test. Desferrioxamine 40 mg/kg in 100 ml normal saline is infused over a 2 hour period 4 hours after dialysis. A base line aluminium of >7.4 μmol/1 (>200 μg/l) or a rise of >7.4 mol/l (200 μg/l) with a normal PTH level 24 hours after infusion is highly suggestive of aluminium intoxication.

Dialysis dementia occurs as a progressive neurological disease to either to aluminium toxicity or multiple cerebral infarcts.

Pruritus

Pruritus is a disabling symptom of uncertain aetiology occurring both on dialysis and between dialyses. There is an association with hyperphosphataemia. Treatment is aimed at:
- reducing plasma phosphate levels
- use of emulsifying creams
- antihistamines (e.g. chlorpheniramine)
- ultraviolet light

Infections

Patients on dialysis are subject to infection, including septicaemia, soft-tissue infections, and tuberculosis. The last may present a difficult diagnostic challenge with pyrexia, atypical lung changes, and abdominal tuberculosis including tuberculous peritonitis. The treatment of tuberculosis in patients with renal failure and on dialysis is discussed in Chapter 12.

Rheumatological complications

These include soft-tissue calcification, gout, pseudogout, haemarthroses, septic arthritis, avascular necrosis and carpal tunnel syndrome. Some joint symptoms are manifestations of hyperparathyroidism but patients who have been on dialysis for more than 10 years develop a symmetrical polyarthritis affecting the shoulder, hands, knees and less commonly other joints (dialysis arthropathy) often in association with a carpal tunnel syndrome. Biopsy of synovia and carpal tunnel tissue reveals amyloid derived from β_2 microglobulin. There is no effective treatment; transplantation appears to help the symptoms. Patients on CAPD may be less likely to develop the problem and the use of more permeable dialysers with or without haemofiltration, is under review.

Anaemia

Anaemia remains one of the outstanding problems associated with haemodialysis patients. In most series, the mean haemoglobin and packed cell volume (PCV) (excluding patients with polycystic kidneys) is $7-8$ g/dl and $20-25\%$ respectively. Patients with polycystic kidneys have a haemoglobin of approximately $8-10$ g/dl and a PCV of $25-30\%$. Patients often become symptomatic until the haemoglobin is below 5 g/dl, unless there is a sharp drop from a higher level. Improved exercise tolerance is due to a shift of the oxygen saturation curve to the right.

Assessment

This includes full blood count, red cell indices, serum and red cell folate, serum B_{12}, serum ferritin and, occasionally, bone marrow appearances. Anaemia may be exacerbated by blood loss, infections, operations and hyperparathyroidism. Occult gastro-intestinal blood loss may require endoscopy and barium studies. Some authorities believe that anaemia may be exacerbated by hypersplenism and corrected by splenectomy.

Treatment

The treatment of the anaemia of chronic renal failure has been revolutionized by the introduction of recombinant DNA erythropoietin. The route and dose of erythropoietin have yet to be fully established but a dose of $50-100$ u/kg $\times$ 3 per week i.v. post dialysis for haemodialysis patients and 50 u/kg × 3 per week subcutaneously for patients on CAPD is currently used. The dose is adjusted to maintain haemoglobin to between $10-11$ g/dl. Side-effects include hypertension, fits and clotted fistulae but may be avoided by controlling blood pressure and raising the haemoglobin levels slowly. All patients should have regular measurements of ferritin levels to assess iron deficiency; iron supplements may be necessary. Occassionally severe iron overload may be treated by a combination of erythropoietin and venesection.

Psychological adaptation to dialysis

Maintenance haemodialysis causes stress to even the most well-adjusted patient and family. Support from medical, technical, nursing and social staff is essential if the patient is to come to terms with his disability. There are financial, social and sexual problems to be faced, all of which require a sympathetic ear and good counselling.

Despite these disadvantages, most patients on haemodialysis adapt remarkably well. Psychiatric problems may be encountered with young patients and with patients dialysing alone. It is invaluable to have access to a sympathetic psychiatrist.

Home dialysis

Although policies of choosing the most suitable form of treatment for patients vary between renal units, the lack of cadaveric kidneys for transplantation, irreversible rejection, age, and failure of peritoneal dialysis, inevitably means that, with the shortage of hospital beds, some patients will require either home or satellite unit dialysis. Home dialysis requires close cooperation between administrative, technical, nursing, social and medical staff. Rooms or cabins are equipped with dialysis machinery familiar to the patient. In general, it takes almost 3 months to train a patient and convert a room for home dialysis.

Follow-up
Patients should be seen every $3-4$ months for review of clinical

status, blood pressure and routine haematological and biochemical tests and should have a full skeletal survey once a
year.

Causes of death
The commonest cause of death is cardiac arrest and myocardial
infarction, followed by cerebrovascular accidents, hyperkalaemia, malignancies and infections.

7.5 Continuous ambulatory peritoneal dialysis (CAPD)

Intermittent peritoneal dialysis has been practised for a number
of years mainly to treat patients before haemodialysis or
transplantation. The results were not impressive, mainly because of infections and inadequate dialysis. However, modern
automated IPD machines give adequate dialysis.

Continuous ambulatory peritoneal dialysis is an attractive
alternative since clearances were increased (especially 'middle
molecule' clearances) with improvement in the patient's general
well-being, anaemia, hypertesion, and easier control of volume
overload. CAPD may be particularly suitable for the elderly,
those with cardiac problems, diabetes and with access problems.

Technique

Catheters
Two types of catheters are now available (Tenchkoff and
Oreopoulos). Tenchkoff catheters may be inserted via a mini
laparotomy or over a guide wire in the ward, whereas
Oreopoulos catheters which are stitched in the pelvis require a
formal laparotomy in theatre. In both procedures antibiotic
cover (Flucloxacillin 250 mg q.d.s., Cefuroxime 750 mg b.d. for
3 days or Vancomycin 1 g i.v. by one dose) is given as prophylaxis. Some units allow the catheters to remain in place 2
weeks before use.

Dialysis
Initially small (0.5 litre) exchanges are used for 48 hours. Thereafter a gradually lengthening dwell time is started so that after 7−10 days 4 or 5 exchanges of 1−2 litres (depending on body size) are made each day. Dialysis solutions contain either 1.36% or 3.86% glucose. Most patients use only 1.36% exchanges and keep an optimum weight by moderating their fluid intake. Occasionally one exchange per day of 3.86% glucose (high osmolar dialysate) is required to maintain optimum weight in a patient with poor fluid compliance. It is inadvisable to exceed more than one exchange of 3.86% glucose because of hyperglycaemia and abnormal blood lipids.

Patients are trained to undertake exchanges using a strict aseptic technique. A 100 g protein diet is encouraged to combat dialysis protein losses (approximately 20 g per day). Fluid restriction is governed by urine output and dialysis ultrafiltration. Patients are taught to measure daily weights, blood pressure, and cumulative dialysate balance. Supplementary vitamin and iron are usually given together with intermittent aluminium hydroxide or calcium carbonate to control phosphate absorption. *The success of a CAPD programme depends on energetic, motivated, nursing staff who train and supervise patients from the moment the catheter is inserted.*

Complications

Peritonitis
This is the most serious complication and should be preventable by thorough training in aseptic techniques. Organisms include:
• coagulase negative staphylococci (75%) from faulty bag exchange techniques or tunnel infections
• Gram-negative organisms sometimes associated with diverticular disease
• other organisms including fungi and mycobacterium tuberculosis

Patients complain of abdominal pain, fever and cloudy dialysate. Examination reveals fever and abdominal tenderness.

Treatment. The treatment for peritonitis involves:
• 3−4 rapid exchanges

• the administration of appropriate antibiotics as in Table 7.4

Table 7.4 Treatment of CAPD peritonitis: antibiotic dosages.

Antibiotic	Loading dose*	Maintenance dose
Tobramycin	1.7 mg/kg i.p.	6 mg/l i.p. (4 mg/l if weight < 60 kg)
Amikacin	6 mg/kg i.p.	6 mg/l i.p.
Cefuroxime	750 mg/l i.p.	250 mg/l i.p.
Ceftazidime	500 mg/l i.p.	125 mg/l i.p.
Ampicillin	250 mg/l i.p.	50 mg/l i.p.
Piperacillin	4 g i.v.	4 g i.v. b.d.
Vancomycin	1 g i.p.	30 mg/l i.p.
Ciprofloxacin	250 mg q.d.s. orally	250 mg q.d.s. orally
Rifampicin	600 mg orally	600 mg o.d.
Amphotericin		0.5 mg/l i.p.
Flucytosine	100 mg/l i.p.	50–100 mg/l i.p.
Fluconazole	400 mg orally	400 mg orally daily
Miconazole		50 mg/l i.p.
Metronidazole		400 mg t.d.s. orally or i.v.

* If i.p. given into first exchange after three quick flushes

The choice of antibiotics depends on local renal unit practices. The following schedules have worked well in practice.

1 Send dialysate to laboratory for gram stains, culture and sensitivity.

2 Give three rapid exchanges.

3 First infection ciprofloxacin 250 mg q.d.s. and vancomycin IG IP. If organism is Gram-negative continue ciprofloxacin until sensitivities are known. If the organism is Gram-positive, stop ciprofloxacin and continue vancomycin for a further two doses at weekly intervals.

4 Other antibiotics and their doses are shown in Table 7.4.

Fungal peritonitis
Fungal peritonitis is often slow and difficult to clear by antifungal agents such as 5-flucytosine, amphotericin B or fluconazole may be effective.

Persistent infections may result in anorexia and excessive protein loss. In these circumstances it is better to discontinue peritoneal dialysis, remove the catheter and haemodialyse the patient short or long term.

Various measures designed to reduce the incidence of peritonitis have been described. These include UV light, and 'heat-seal' sterilization, and of most importance is the use of 'Y cut' lines.

Technical and mechanical complications
Catheters may be poorly sited, drain poorly or leak. Sudden cessation of outflow may be caused by omentum wrapping around the catheter tip and may be corrected by ambulation and relief of constipation. Leakage from catheter implant site may be helped by reducing the volume of dialysis fluid with shorter dwell times.

Other complications
Repeated episodes of peritonitis may lead to loss of peritoneal function. The peritoneum may sclerose for no apparent reason. Hyperglycaemia and hypertriglyceridaemia may occur. Backache is a common complaint.

Results

It is too early to judge the long-term outcome of patients on CAPD. Many patients feel better, have higher haemoglobin and prefer CAPD to haemodialysis. Some, however, dislike the monotony of 4 or 5 daily exchanges, the presence of a catheter, the risk of infection, and request to return to haemodialysis. Results of haemodialysis, CAPD and transplantation survival are shown in Table 7.5.

7.6 Transplantation

Kidneys may be transplanted from either a relative (parents or siblings, occasionally children or others) or a cadaver. In Britain the number of kidney donors does not match the demand

Table 7.5 Percentage of patient survival on various treatment modalities.

Type and length of treatment	Age (years)		
	15−44	45−64	> 65
Haemodialysis			
5 years	76	58	35
10 years	52	23	7
CAPD			
4 years	74	54	30
Primary renal disease			
5 years	79	60	34
Diabetic nephropathy			
5 years	44	25	13
5 years following transplant	83	67	53

Modified from Brunner *et al.* (1988) *Nephrol. Dial. Transplant* **2**: 109−122

and the list of potential recipients is gradually increasing (over 3500 in 1989).

Selection and preparation of recipient

There are very few contraindications for transplantation although patients with malignant disease, severe atheromatous disease (recent stroke or myocardial infarction), and those aged over 70 years, are unlikely to be included in many centres on a transplant list.

Preparation
Preparation of recipient includes:
- recent chest X-ray and hand X-rays
- gastroscopy and anti-ulcer therapy if indicated
- blood group and tissue type
- bilateral nephrectomy in patients with very large polycystic kidneys, renal malignancies or severe infection
- parathyroidectomy for severe hyperparathyroidism

Most patients are on dialysis but pre-dialysis patients have been successfully transplanted.

Tissue typing

Histocompatibility (HLA) antigens are located in chromosome 6 and comprise of four known loci A, B, C, and DR. In practice typing for A, B and DR is undertaken. Each locus has two alleles and as the number of antigens amount to 30–40 at each locus, an immense number of genotypes is possible. There is evidence that a 'full house' (2A, 2B and 2DR) has a better graft survival than lesser A and B matches and also some evidence that 2DR matches have superior graft survival rates than 1 or 0, DR matches. However immunosuppression with Cyclosporin and anti-thymocyte globulin has resulted in superior results and many transplant units are using kidneys with donors who are ABO compatible only.

Anti-lymphocyte antibodies may be found in the sera of recipients as a result of previous transplants, blood transfusions or pregnancy. Recipients vary from nil antibodies to having antibodies against all panel donor antigens. These latter patients may be difficult to transplant and attempts are being made to find ways of reducing the antibody level; for example by immunoabsorption.

Direct cross-match

A positive T cell cross-match using the current serum precludes transplantation. Positive T cell cross-matches from previous sera or positive B cell cross-matches may be ignored.

Transplants outside of ABO compatibilities

Transplantation follows normal blood transfusion principles. It has also been found that blood group A1 (but not A2) kidneys may be transplanted into O recipients. Other blood group mismatches result in hyperacute rejection.

Red cell antibodies

Multiple red cell antibodies (especially Lewis antibodies) may be of importance to transplant survival.

Preparation of donor

Living related donors
These may be either parents; siblings; children or rarely, unrelated donors including spouses. Selection should be based on tissue typing, physical fitness and psychological adaptation. There are ethical problems if children under the age of 25 are used as donors. Parents (or children) will share 1 haplotype, siblings none, 1 or 2 haplotypes. A detailed history should be established and the following investigations should be carried out prior to transplantation.
- FBC, blood group and tissue type
- urea, electrolytes, creatinine, creatinine clearance or ^{51}Cr EDTA clearance, calcium, phosphate, liver function tests and glucose
- MSU, hepatitis antigen and cytomegalovirus (CMV) titre
- IVP, renogram, ultrasound, arteriogram, including selective renal arteriogram and chest X-ray

Special problems
- some authorities suggest that a glucose tolerance test is undertaken on donors of patients with diabetes
- special care should be taken in evaluating donor kidneys in children whose parents have polycystic kidneys
- motivation is of such importance that some units refer potential kidney donors for a psychiatric opinion

Cadaver donors
The *Human Tissue Act* of 1986 allows viable kidneys to be removed from beating heart donors provided that certain criteria are fulfilled, (see Appendix 7).

Most potential cadaver donors present as a result of road traffic accidents, self-poisoning or primary intracranial disorders, such as a subarachnoid haemorrhage or a primary intracranial tumour. Patients with widespread malignancies, or infections, those older than 65, or those who have had long periods of hypotension, are generally unsuitable as donors.

The *warm ischaemic time* is the time taken from switching off the resuscitator equipment to perfusing the kidneys with cooled physiological fluid (e.g. Collins or Marshalls fluid). The *cold ischaemic time* is the time from kidney perfusion until insertion into the recipient. Ideally, the warm ischaemic time should not exceed 60 minutes and the cold ischaemic time 24 hours, but kidneys with cold ischaemic times of up to 72 hours have been successfully transplanted.

Technique of transplantation

The kidney is transplanted in an extraperitoneal site in the iliac fossa. The renal artery is anastomosed end to end with the internal iliac artery and the renal vein end to side with either the common or external iliac vein. The donor ureter may be anastomosed to the bladder or ureter of the recipient. Some units give antibiotics and/or dopamine perioperatively and use stents to prevent ureteric obstruction.

Immunosuppressive therapy

The introduction of cyclosporin A, antithymocyte globulin (ATG) and more specific T cell antibody preparations (such as OKT3) has radically changed immunosuppressive therapy. Unfortunately there are many different policies but most are based on cyclosporin as the principle immunosuppressive agent. The following schemes are under evaluation.

Single drug therapy
Cyclosporin alone is used as the sole immunosuppressive drug.

Double drug therapy
Cyclosporin is used in combination with prednisolone or azathioprine.

Triple drug therapy
There are two types of immunosuppression therapy under this heading.
1 Triple therapy from the start of transplantation using cyclosporin, prednisolone and azathioprine.

2 Sequential therapy using ATG, prednisolone and azathio-prine until diuresis occurs when ATG is substituted by cy-closporin. In patients who diurese from the start ATG is given for 5 days only. ATG is replaced by cyclosporin at 14 days if a diuresis has not commenced.

Details of doses are usually worked out a local level. The aim of triple therapy is to minimize the risk of toxicity of each drug by reducing the dose to a minimum. In well functioning kidneys by day 14, the dose of cyclosporin should be ap-proximately 3−4 mg/kg/day giving trough cyclosporin levels of 60−160 ng/ml (depending on method of assay); prednisolone 15 mg/day and azathioprine 1 mg/kg/day.

Most transplant units use double or triple drug therapy with claims of 90% cadaver graft function at one year using sequential therapy.

Newer drugs

Newer drugs are likely to be introduced as immunosuppressive agents, including FK506, which is currently under evaluation. There are controversies concerning the use of cyclosporin A.

1 The use in non-diuresing kidneys where some authorities advocate substituting either azathioprine or ATG until a diuresis result.

2 Switching from cyclosporin A to azathioprine at 3, 6 or 12 months post-transplant in order to avoid long-term nephrotoxicity.

3 The type of assay (? monoclonal ? polyclonal) or HPLC to measure levels. Most transplant units measure trough whole blood levels using a radioimmunoassay technique.

Side-effects of cyclosporin include:
- nephrotoxicity which is dose related and usually reversible (avoided by keeping whole blood trough levels under 200 ng/ml)
- tremor and rarely grand mal seizures
- hirsutism
- venous thromboses
- various drug interactions (see p. 199)

Rejection

Hyperacute
This occurs within the first 24 hours of transplantation and is due to recipient preformed antibodies reacting with donor kidney tissue. It should be avoided by correct ABO matching and a negative direct lymphocyte cross-match. There is no treatment for hyperacute rejection. The kidney shows widespread thromboses.

Acute
Acute rejection occurs within 1 week to 1 year of transplantation but is most frequent from 2 weeks to 2 months. Clinical signs of acute rejection include fever, graft pain and tenderness, fluid retention and hypertension. There is sodium retention, proteinuria and a falling GFR. Biopsy shows either a widespread cellular infiltrate (cellular rejection) or endothelial swelling and thromboses (vascular rejection).

Numerous tests have been described to confirm the diagnosis of rejection: none are totally satisfactory. Doppler ultrasound reveals cortical blood flow patterns and may give early evidence of acute rejection. Isotope renography defines the vascular supply and serial perfusion indices may also give evidence of rejection.

Other test of rejection have included intrarenal pressures, urinary enzymes, use of radiolabelled platelets and fine needle aspiration. Many believe however that the 'gold standard' in diagnosis is a renal biopsy. This is particularly true in the first week of transplantation when rejection may be superimposed on acute tubular necrosis. Differential diagnoses of acute rejection within the first 4 weeks of transplantation are shown in Table 7.6.

Chronic
This is largely a vascular process with marked inflammatory changes in medium size arteries and arterioles. There is no known treatment.

Management of rejection

Traditionally acute rejection has been treated with methyl-prednisolone (500 mg or 1 g i.v.) bolus × 3, but smaller doses have been claimed to be equally effective. Solumedrone must be given slowly over 15 minutes. Most units limit the number of courses to 2 or 3. If the kidney continues to show cellular rejection (steroid resistant rejection) either ATG (3 mg/kg daily or OKT_3 5 mg daily i.v.) may be given over 10−14 days. Both drugs have to be given after a negative test dose. Both may result in fever and general malaise. Patients given OKT_3 must not be fluid overloaded. Both drugs are extremely expensive.

Acute vascular rejection is difficult to treat but all the above measures and occasionally plasmaphoresis are sometimes effective.

Follow-up of transplant patients

During the initial period after transplantation, a combined urology and nephrology policy of patient care is essential, involving twice daily ward rounds. Daily blood tests for blood count, platelets, urea, electrolytes, creatinine and glucose levels, three times a week for calcium and phosphate levels, liver function tests, amylase, and once a week MSU, CMV titres and chest X-ray (CXR), are required.

The first 2−3 weeks post-transplant are the most anxious time for patient and staff alike. Cadaver grafts may not 'open up' for 2 weeks or more and many patients experience 1 or 2 rejection episodes. Careful monitoring of fluid balance, patient weight, blood count, electrolyte, glucose, suture lines, as well as renal function, are mandatory.

Other drugs post-transplant

In addition to immunosuppressive agents, many units also give an antacid, e.g. Asilone 10 ml t.d.s. and ranitidine 150 daily to protect the oesophageal and gastric mucosa and nystatin suspension 100 000 u (1 ml) q.d.s. as a prophylaxis against candida, during the time of high steroid dosage. Some

Table 7.6 Differential diagnosis of acute rejection of kidney transplant.

Event	Clinical signs	Confirmatory test	Treatment
Acute tubular necrosis	Oliguria after transplant	Biopsy	Wait for recovery, avoid nephrotoxic agents
Acute obstruction	Oliguria, occasional extravasation, worsening renal function	Renography, ultrasound, exploration	Surgery
Acute arterial insufficiency	Oliguria, worsening renal function	Renography, arteriography, exploration	Surgery
Acute infection	Fever, tender kidney	Urinary infection, MSU	Antibiotics

units also give acyclovir as a prophylaxis against herpes
infections.

Follow-up after discharge

In the first 2−3 months very careful follow-up is required,
with weekly monitoring of renal function, blood count, weight,
blood pressure and urine cultures. In general, patients are
seen weekly for 1 month, every 2 weeks for a further 2 months
and then monthly for 6 months.

7.7 Complications of renal transplantation

Early surgical complications include ureteric leaks; ureteric
stenoses; blocked catheters and, rarely, leaking or blocked
vascular anastomoses. Lymphatic fluid may collect near the
kidney as a *lymphocoele*, and this can be of sufficient size to
obstruct urine flow. Lymphocoeles are best demonstrated by
ultrasound and may be treated by aspiration and the instillation
of radioactive colloidal gold.

Gastro-intestinal haemorrhage

This may be a catastrophic acute bleed from a large duodenal
ulcer or lesser degrees of bleeding from gastric erosions.
Pretransplant endoscopy (if clinically indicated) and use of
ranitidine should prevent serious gastro-intestinal bleeding.

Long-term complications

All transplant patients suffer from the risks of developing
complications secondary to long-term immunosuppression.

Infections
These are summarized as in Table 7.7.

Side-effects of azathioprine
These include bone-marrow depression, especially leucopenia,
thrombocytopenia and anaemia. Persistent leucopenia with

Table 7.7 Infections after kidney transplantation.

Infection	Organism	Treatment
Septicaemia	Gram-positive cocci Gram-negative bacilli Anaerobic organisms	Aminoglycoside + flucloxacillin + metronidazole or ceftazidine + metronidaxole
Bacterial infection of skin, lung, urinary tract, meninges, joints or bone	As identified	Relevant to organism
Herpes infection	Herpes simplex Herpes zoster	Local idoxuridine or acyclovir orally or i.v.
Other viruses	Cytomegalovirus Epstein–Barr	Gangcyclovir or Foscarnet for severe infection No treatment available
Protozoal infection	Pneumocystis carinii	Cotrimoxazole or pyrimethamine + sulphadiazine
Fungal infection Generalized	Candida albicans C. tropicalis Torulopsis glabrata Coccidiomycosis (and others)	Fluconazole or amphoteracin B or flucytosine
Localized	Candida	Nystatin
Tuberculosis	Mycobacterium tuberculosis	Antituberculous chemotherapy

relatively low doses of azathioprine may require either splenectomy or a change to cyclophosphamide or cyclosporin.

Side-effects of steroids affecting the skin

These are Cushingoid appearances, acne and bruising.

Bone complications

Avascular necrosis occurs in approximately 20–30% of a transplant population, particularly in those with pre-existing hyperparathyroidism, and it affects weight-bearing joints, especially the hips and knees. Confirmation is by X-ray and treatment usually necessitates joint replacement.

Hyperparathyroidism will be present to varying extents at the time of transplantation unless a total parathyroidectomy has been carried out within a year or 2 of transplantation. In most cases the release of endogenous 1-25 vitamin D_3 from the transplanted kidney is sufficient to suppress PTH production. In some patients hypercalcaemia may occur, requiring either parathyroidectomy or medical treatment with, for example, frusemide and Slow sodium to induce a calcium diuresis (see p. 38).

Osteoporosis may occur as a result of long-term steroid administration. The only effective treatment is to reduce steroid dosage, preferably with an alternate-day regimen.

Failure to grow is the primary abnormality in children. It may be minimized by alternate-day doses of steroids.

Hypertension

Many transplant patients suffer with hypertension which can be controlled by calcium channel blockers and diuretics. Care must be taken not to dehydrate patients for fear of compromising renal function.

Renal artery stenosis

Renal artery stenosis is a rare complication of renal transplantation and may present with either worsening renal function or hypertension. Diagnosis may be made by renography (with and without captopril) or angiography. Treatment may be attempted by angioplasty or surgical reanastomosis.

Acute pancreatitis
This may be fatal, and occurs in about 2% of all transplant patients.

Psychiatric complications
These are not infrequent. All varieties of affective disorders may be seen, ranging from euphoria to depression, including frank steroid psychoses. Some patients exhibit 'machine-dependency' syndrome, appearing to prefer the rigours of dialysis to the freedom of transplantation. Close psychiatric cooperation is required for the well-being of these patients.

Hepatitis
Hepatitis is occasionally associated with azathioprine therapy. Most transplanted patients have high mean cell volumes without abnormal liver function tests.

Development of neoplasms
Epithelial tumours of the skin including the lip, carcinoma of the cervix and mesenchymal tumours, especially lymphomas, occur more frequently in transplanted patients than in age-matched control subjects. Lymphomas are particularly interesting since they metastasise to the brain or spinal cord. Careful inspection of the skin and regular cervical smears would seem appropriate. The lymphomas may be difficult to treat without stopping immunosuppressives.

Results

The European Dialysis and Transplant Association–European Renal Association regularly reports on patient and graft survival. Some representative data for transplants undertaken between 1980 and 1984 are shown in Table 7.8. It should be noted that there is considerable inter-transplant unit variation and the results for graft survival are disappointingly low for some categories.

Causes of death

Septicaemia remains the most common cause of death among transplant patients, followed by arterial disease (myocardial infarction, cerebrovascular disease) and in older patients, pulmonary embolism. Other infections, gastro-intestinal haemorrhage, pancreatitis and malignancy, are also important causes.

Table 7.8 5-year graft and patient survival in Europe, 1980−84 (%).

	Age at grafting (years)	
	15−44	45−64
1st cadaver		
Graft survival	51	46
Patient survival	83	67
Living related		
Graft survival	66	60
Patient survival	87	72
2nd cadaver		
Graft survival	47	
Patient survival	85	61

Brunner *et al.* (1988) *Nephrol. Dial. Transplant* **3**: 109−122

Conclusion

The lessons of earlier experience are gradually being learned about transplantation. For it to be successful, adequate preparation of the donor, optimum (preferably DR) matching, and low-dose steroids, are needed. Modern immunosuppression with triple therapy appear to be enhancing graft survival.

8: Urinary infection and X-ray abnormalities

8.1 Introduction

These conditions are considered together since they share certain clinical features, e.g. loin pain and symptomatic urinary infections. Reflux, analgesic and obstructive nephropathy, may also be confused radiologically.

Urinary tract infections are among the most common conditions seen in nephrological practice. Precise definitions are important since a great deal of misunderstanding in diagnosis and management may occur if imprecision is allowed.

Definitions

Bacteriuria
This is the presence of viable or living organism in the bladder urine. There may, or may not, be symptoms.

'Significant' bacteriuria
This is the presence of a pure growth of $> 10^5$/ml bacteria in an MSU, or any number of bacteria found in urine obtained by supra-pubic aspiration of the bladder.

Urinary tract infection
This is the presence of micro-organisms in the urinary tract. Traditionally, infection implies invasion and inflammation, with or without symptoms.

For other definitions, see respective sections.

8.2 Bacteriology of urinary tract infections

Common organisms causing urinary tract infections include *Escherichia coli*, other Gram-negative organisms (e.g. *Klebsiella*, *Enterobacter*, *Proteus* spp. and *Pseudomonas*), Gram-positive cocci (coagulase negative and positive staphylococci, *Streptococcus faecalis*). Certain other micro-organisms responsible for both lower (bladder) and upper (above the bladder) urinary infections have more recently been described, including mycoplasmas, chlamydiae, and possibly various fastidious organisms formerly thought to be commensals. Most pathogenic organisms are found in normal bowel flora and reach the urinary tract by way of vestibular and urethral colonization. The mechanisms whereby bladder or renal infections become established is often unclear but involve the failure of normal defence mechanisms (including structural abnormalities of the urinary tract) as well as certain bacterial characteristics, e.g. serotype and the presence of bacterial pili associated with adhesiveness.

The collection and bacterial quantitation of urine cultures have added to the understanding of the epidemiology of urinary tract infections, but need careful interpretation. Table 8.1 sets out a guide of the number of bacteria in normal and infected urine together with the number of red and white cells found.

In clinical practice, urinary infection may present in five ways: asymptomatic bacteriuria, acute cystitis, acute pyelonephritis, reflux nephropathy, and infection secondary to structural damage of the urinary tract.

8.3 Asymptomatic bacteriuria

This is significant bacteriuria without symptoms. It is generally used as an epidemiological term although 'covert bacteriuria' is preferred by some. Population screening has been undertaken in the following three groups.

Children
The prevalence of bacteriuria in girls aged 5 is about 1%. Extensive studies have not shown that treating girls with asymptomatic bacteriuria reduces the incidence of renal scarring or renal failure. Screening pre-school infants for reflux might be of benefit if some suitable test could be devised.

Pregnant women
The prevalence of bacteriuria in the first trimester is about 5% in Caucasian women. Treatment of bacteriuria in pregnancy

Table 8.1 Urine culture findings.

		Quantitative culture: bacteria per ml	White blood cells per mm^3	Red blood cells per mm^3
Not infected	MSU	$<10^4$	<10	<10
	SPA	Sterile	Not defined	Not defined
	CSU	$<10^4$	<10	<10
Infected	MSU	$>10^5(\times 2)$	$<$ or >10	$<$ or >10
	SPA	Any number	Not defined	Not defined
	CSU	$>10^5$	$<$ or >10	$<$ or >10

MSU: mid-stream urine sample; SPA: suprapubic aspiration urine sample; CSU: catheter sample of urine.
NB
1 Bacteriuria may be present in an MSU or CSU with bacterial counts of $<10^3$ or $<10^4$/ml if a pure growth is present.
2 The presence of excess white cells may indicate inflammation rather than infections. Acute symptomatic urinary tract infections are usually associated with white cells in excess of 50/mm^3.
3 Only suprapubic aspiration of the bladder can be certain to accurately assess bacteriuria.

substantially reduces the incidence of subsequent symptomatic upper urinary tract infections and possibly reduces the incidence of prematurity and fetal malformation. Investigation post-partum reveals a number of women (20–30% of those with bacteriuria) who have some underlying urinary tract abnormality. Screening for bacteriuria in pregnancy should therefore be established in obstetric practice.

Adult non-pregnant women aged 20–50
This group shows a prevalence of bacteriuria of about 4%. There is no convincing evidence that treating bacteriuria in non-pregnant adults is of any value. Adult patients with asymptomatic bacteriuria rarely develop symptomatic bacteriuria, further renal scars, or worsening renal function.

8.4 Acute bacterial cystitis ('posterior urethritis', 'frequency and dysuria syndrome of bacterial origin')

Acute cystitis is the commonest urinary infection seen in clinical (particularly general) practice. Symptoms include frequency, dysuria, lower abdominal pain, backache, occasionally loin pain, but not tenderness or fever. Symptoms suggestive of bacterial cystitis may occur with other pathological processes and may be incorporated into the general term 'urethral syndrome' (frequency and dysuria syndrome). Some other causes of the urethral syndrome are as follows:
- other causes of urethritis/cystitis e.g. non-specific urethritis (NSU), gonococci, tuberculosis of the bladder, interstitial cystitis, cystitis due to drugs, e.g. cyclophosphamide
- urethral/bladder stones, urethral/bladder tumours, urethral polyps
- vaginitis (chemical, trichomonas, *Candida*), cervical infections, senile vaginitis

As can be seen, the conditions mimicking cystitis are diverse and it is therefore important that patients who have 'bacterial' cystitis should be investigated.

Microbiology

E. coli are found in 70% of cases, coagulase negative staphylococci (strictly micrococci) in 25%, other organisms (*Streptococcus faecalis*, other Gram-negative organisms) in 5%. The bacteriology of bacterial cystitis has been extended to include chlamydiae, mycoplasmas (possibly), and organisms long regarded as commensal, e.g. diphtheroids and corynebacteria. These so called 'fastidious' organisms are difficult to culture in routine hospital microbiological departments.

The treatment of these different organisms is shown in Table 8.2. Note that most acute lower urinary infections can be treated by a *single or double dose* of amoxycillin or co-trimoxazole similar in principle to the treatment of gonorrhoea.

Table 8.2 Treatment of bacterial cystitis.

Causative organism	Treatment
E. coli Micrococci	Amoxycillin 3 g b.d. (with 6-hour interval) or co-trimoxazole 4 tabs, 2 doses (with 6-hour interval) or trimethoprim 100 mg b.d. or nitrofurantoin 50 mg q.d.s. or ampicillin 500 mg t.d.s. for 5 days
Mycoplasma Chlamydiae	Tetracycline 250 mg q.d.s. for one week
Fastidious organism	Amoxycillin or erythromycin

Recurrent infections

Some women suffer with recurrent cystitis. Attempts to reduce the attacks by such measures as perineal hygiene, bathing, double micturition, etc., may help but the use of long-term low-dose antibiotics such as nitrofurantoin (50 mg), trimethoprim (100 mg) or cephalexin (125 mg) has been proved to be extremely effective. Treatment should continue for 6–12 months. Patients with recurrent cystitis, or who have associated heavy haematuria, need investigation including a urogram with or without cystoscopy.

8.5 Acute pyelonephritis

This condition usually develops from untreated acute bacterial cystitis, and consists of loin pain and tenderness, fever and bacteriuria. There are usually lower urinary symptoms and excess urinary white and, occasionally, red blood cells. Complications include bacteraemia and septicaemia. In some patients, the disease is mild, others may be severely ill with rigors, anorexia, severe pain and shock.

Treatment consists of the administration of some suitable antimicrobial agent which achieves adequate blood and urine levels, e.g. co-trimoxazole, ampicillin, or a cephalosporin. Severely ill patients with septicaemia require treatment with an aminoglycoside, e.g. tobramycin. Treatment should continue for 2 weeks.

Patients with acute pyelonephritis admitted to hospital require (in addition to more routine tests):
- a pregnancy test
- plain X-ray of the abdomen — to visualize renal outlines and renal or ureteric stones
- ultrasound — to exclude obstruction
- blood culture, blood count and renal function
- occasionally, an 'emergency' IVU (if urinary obstruction is suspected)

All patients with acute pyelonephritis should have an IVU or ultrasound (at some stage) to exclude some structural abnormality of the urinary tract.

Differential diagnosis

Acute pyelonephritis can resemble other renal conditions (renal colic, loin pain and haematuria syndrome), other abdominal problems (cholecystitis, appendicitis, salpingitis and other pelvic problems) and even extra-abdominal pathologies, e.g. pneumonia. Rapid evaluation of the urine, is vital to avoid an unnecessary laparotomy.

Follow-up

Follow-up of patients with acute pyelonephritis is essential
since 50% of patients will relapse within 6 months. Low-dose
prophylactic chemotherapy is equally successful in controlling
recurrent acute pyelonephritis, as for acute cystitis (see above),
unless there is some major structural abnormality of the urinary
tract (e.g. renal calculus).

8.6 Reflux nephropathy

This term has now replaced the antiquated 'chronic
pyelonephritis' which has variable clinical, bacteriological,
histological and radiological implications. Reflux nephropathy
is defined by radiological appearance and corresponds to what
was at one time called 'primary atrophic pyelonephritis'.

Reflux nephropathy originates in infancy (possibly *in utero*?)
and is due to vesico ureteric and intra-renal reflux. The damage
to papillae may be localized to one or both kidneys and may
affect one, several, or all of the papillae. In children, reflux
nephropathy is associated with failure to thrive, recurrent
symptomatic urinary tract infections and, rarely, renal failure
or hypertension. In adults, patients may be subject to symptomatic urinary tract infections, renal stones, hypertension
and, rarely, impaired renal function. Renal failure is more
likely to occur in patients with heavy (>2 g 24 hours)
proteinuria which is indicative of superimposed glomerular
damage (focal sclerosis). The radiological differential diagnosis
is shown in Figure 8.1, and includes the following.

1 Obstructive nephropathy (or uropathy, hydronephrosis) (see
p. 158).

2 Papillary necrosis (see p. 157).

3 Persistent fetal lobulation.

4 Calyceal cysts — benign fluid-filled cavities usually connected
to the calyx by a channel. They may calcify or become infected,
but rarely require treatment other than antibiotics for symptomatic infection.

5 Tuberculosis of the urinary tract must never be forgotten. It
often presents insidiously and, unless early morning urine

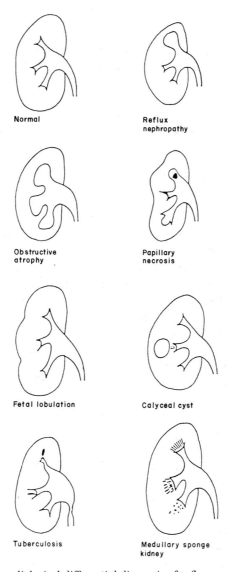

Fig. 8.1 The radiological differential diagnosis of reflux nephropathy.

samples for tuberculosis bacilli are requested for even minor abnormalities of the urinary tract, and for sterile pyuria, cases will go undiagnosed. Treatment follows traditional lines of tuberculosis elsewhere in the body, but careful follow-up radiology is required since obstruction and a 'medical nephrectomy' may follow.

6 Medullary sponge kidney is a fairly common condition and is discussed under cystic lesion of the kidney (p. 162).

Management

Severe degrees of reflux in a young child should be corrected by reimplantation of the ureter and careful follow-up to anticipate and treat urinary tract infections, whether symptomatic or not. Lesser degrees of reflux may be left, particularly in older children, since there is a tendency for the reflux to disappear with maturity. Prompt treatment of infection is mandatory and a case can be made for long-term low-dose prophylactic treatment, e.g. with co-trimoxazole paed one tablet at night, trimethoprim paed suspension 50 mg at night or cephalexin suspension 125 mg at night (all doses appropriate for age and size), until the age of 12 or 13. Regular follow-up is required with repeat urine cultures.

In adults, surgery may, rarely, be required to repair severe degrees of reflux, but repeat cystograms are advisable after a course of treatment for any infection since reflux may improve in adults, with treatment. Rarely, a nephrectomy may be required where the kidney is contributing to less than 20% of overall total renal function. The principles of treatment of infections are similar to those of patients with a normal urogram: eradication of upper urinary infection with a 7–14 day course of antibiotics followed by long-term, low-dose prophylactic treatment if recurrent infections are frequent.

8.7 Infections in patients with renal stones, catheter and paraplegia

The following three areas represent the most difficult to treat of all types of patients who have urinary tract infections.

Renal stones

Patients with renal stones (Chapter 10) may have urinary infections which are impossible to eradicate until the stone is removed. The urine may be rendered sterile which, in theory, may prevent further stone growth. Long-term treatment (with larger doses of antibiotics than is used for prophylaxis) may be used, and also following removal of 'triple phosphate' staghorn calculi, to prevent fresh stones forming.

Catheters

These present a particular challenge since the art lies in prevention rather than treatment. Catheterization is undertaken using a strict aseptic technique and utilizing a closed drainage system. Daily meatal toilet and aspiration from sites on the catheter without breaking catheter continuity will help to prevent infections. The use of antibiotic bladder wash-outs has not been shown to reduce the development of infection and may precipitate infection with highly resistant organisms. Catheters need only to be changed if drainage is inadequate.

Paraplegia

Patients with paraplegia develop (almost uniquely) renal failure associated with scarred kidneys and infection if long-term catheters are used for bladder drainage. Strict aseptic intermittent catheterization has some advantage, but ideally the patient should be taught twice a day *bladder expression*. The urine should be regularly cultured for infection and urograms obtained at 2-yearly intervals. In the event of difficulty controlling infections or the occurrence of radiological damage, reimplantation of the ureter into an ileal conduit should be considered.

Localization of urinary tract infection

Various techniques have been described to determine the site of urinary tract infections. These include urinary enzyme tests, ureteric catheterization, the bladder wash-out technique, serum antibodies and, an immunofluorescent technique utilizing the fact that bacteria from 'upper' (above the bladder) urinary infections are coated with antibody whereas bacteria from 'lower' (bladder or below) urinary infections are not coated.

Localization of infections may be useful in deciding the best method of treatment since it has been postulated that an upper urinary infection requires longer treatment with anti- biotics achieving adequate blood and urine levels than a lower urinary infection. However, all localization procedures have unacceptably high false-negative and false-positive results and at present may indicate tissue invasion rather than local- ization. They are not widely used in clinical practice.

8.8 Urinary infection in men

Below the age of 70, urinary infections in men occur less frequently than women but thereafter increase due to prostatic hypertrophy. Asymptomatic infections in young men are very unusual. Symptomatic infections may originate from the pro- state and spread to the testes, epididymis or kidneys. Prostatic infections are difficult to diagnose and require treatment with tetracyclines, erythromycin or co-trimoxazole which penetrates prostatic tissue rather than lactam antibiotics.

The prevalence of urinary tract abnormalities is high among men with urinary infection due to aerobic organisms and justi- fies simple investigation such as plain X-ray of the abdomen and ultrasound. Elderly institutionalized men tend to develop urinary tract infection and need not be treated unless they become symptomatic or require surgery to the urinary tract.

8.9 Xanthogranulomatous pyelonephritis

This rare condition presents as loin pain and is seen in patients of all ages, predominantly women. Examination may reveal a tender renal mass and investigation shows a non-functioning enlarged kidney with calculi and a urinary infection due to a Proteus organism. Lipid containing cells with some features reminiscent of a hypernephroma are found on histology. Treatment is usually by nephrectomy.

8.10 Renal papillary necrosis

Renal papillary necrosis may be caused by:
- chronic analgesic abuse (especially phenacetin)
- diabetes mellitus
- sickle cell trait
- alcoholism

Analgesic neuropathy may be mistaken for reflux nephropathy since the X-rays bear some superficial similarities. *All* patients with renal disease should be closely questioned about present and past analgesic intake, especially phenacetin-containing drugs. Most patients with analgesic nephropathy are women of about 50 who present with a variety of problems including chronic renal failure, haematuria, dyspepsia, urinary infection, or occasionally with acute-on-chronic renal failure due to either surgery to the gastro-intestinal tract or bilateral obstruction with impacted calcified papillae. Examination shows stigmata of chronic renal failure with a typical personality including obsessional traits, depression, alcoholism and excess smoking. Differentiation from reflux nephropathy is shown in Table 8.3.

Table 8.3 Differentiation of reflux nephropathy and analgesic nephropathy.

Reflux nephropathy	Analgesic nephropathy
May be unilateral or bilateral	Always bilateral
Typical X-ray appearance	Typical X-ray appearance
Renal function usually normal	Renal function often abnormal
Minor degree of lack of concentrating ability	Severe degree of lack of concentrating ability
Reflux present in 50% of bilateral cases	Reflux rare
Prognosis good	Prognosis good providing analgesic intake stopped

Treatment is firstly to withhold analgesics, especially phenacetin, and prostaglandin inhibitors (e.g. indomethacin), since prostaglandin may be important to maintain residual medullary blood flow, especially in the presence of saline loss. Patients with papillary necrosis are especially prone to the ill-effects of dehydration and prophylactic saline is essential to cover surgery. Complications of analgesic nephropathy include:

- anaemia
- carcinoma of renal pelvis, ureteric fibrosis
- peptic ulceration
- neuropsychiatric complications, including dementia

The important point is to remember to ask all patients with renal failure about analgesic consumption. The withdrawal of phenacetin from all tablets should lead to a decline in the incidence of the disease since there is very little evidence that other analgesics can be implicated as a cause of renal damage.

8.11 Obstructive uropathy

Acute
Acute urinary obstruction is considered in Chapter 4.

Chronic
Chronic obstruction is of interest to the nephrologist as a number of different abnormalities of renal function may be found.

1 A reduction in GFR consequent on a raised proximal tubular lumen pressure, fall in renal blood flow and nephron damage. Prolonged (> 7 days) obstruction leads to permanent reduction in GFR and the early relief of obstruction is therefore important.
2 A reduced urine concentrating ability resulting in polyuria and occasionally hypernatraemia.
3 A reduced urinary acidification, unlikely to cause a metabolic acidosis.
4 Hyperkalaemia associated with hyporeninaemic hypoaldosteronism.

The list of possible causes of chronic obstruction is very long, but includes congenital (pelvic-ureteric obstruction, urethral valves), traumatic (e.g. following stone or urethral damage), inflammatory (retroperitoneal fibrosis, tuberculosis) obstruction and tumours (bladder, prostate), stones, and benign prostatic hypertrophy. Many of these conditions are outside the scope of this text but the nephrologist should always be alert to the possibility that acute or chronic obstruction is the cause of the patient's renal problems.

Retroperitoneal fibrosis

This is a rare but important cause of obstruction. The condition affects men more than women and characteristically presents with backache, constipation, vomiting, hydrocoele and, occasionally, oliguria or anuria. The condition is associated with the chronic consumption of certain drugs, notably amphetamines, practolol, methysergide, or with the retroperitoneal spread of tumours. However, the most important association is with aortic aneurysms when slow leakage from the aneurysm results in an inflammatory reaction involving the ureters.

Diagnosis is confirmed by urography or ultrasound which shows the characteristic bilateral hydronephrosis and medial deviation of the ureters. Treatment is either surgical (ureterolysis) or with the use of steroids, e.g. prednisolone 20 mg t.d.s. Surgery offers the advantage of the ability to biopsy the retroperitoneal tissues, but the response to steroids can be very impressive, with a gradually tapering dose so that the course is finished within 3 months.

Retroperitoneal fibrosis can affect the vascular supply to the legs or abdominal viscera and the fibrotic process occasionally spreads to the mediastinum.

8.12 Chronic interstitial nephritis

This is a pathological term used to describe an inflammatory infiltrate of the 'interstitium' of the kidney with secondary changes in the glomeruli, tubules and vessels. There are a number of causes including:
• drugs, e.g. phenacetin (changes secondary to papillary necrosis)
• infections (reflux nephropathy)
• gout
• Sjögren's syndrome

- radiation (mainly interstitial fibrosis)
- Balkan nephropathy (mainly interstitial fibrosis)
- medullary cystic disease (changes secondary to medullary cysts, p. 162)
- hereditary nephritis (p. 167)
- hypertension and renal vascular disease
- paraproteinaemia
- heavy metals

Balkan nephropathy

This is a special form of interstitial nephritis occurring endemically in an area of the Danube and its tributaries in Yugoslavia and Bulgaria. Patients present with mild proteinuria, progressive renal failure or anaemia; oedema and hypertension are unusual. Interstitial fibrosis is found in terminal stages; mild glomerular changes have been described in biopsies from early cases. There is often a family history of the condition. A high incidence of urothelial tumours has been described. The aetiology is unclear: a nephrotoxic mycotoxin from cereal grain has been suggested. There is no known treatment.

Radiation nephritis

Acute and chronic radiation produces interstitial oedema and widespread glomerular, vascular and interstitial degenerative changes, leading to variable degrees of renal damage. Patients present either acutely with hypertension (sometimes malignant), nephrotic syndrome or renal failure, or may follow a more chronic course with chronic renal failure, anaemia or hypertension. There is no known treatment and current practice is to shield the kidneys (especially in children) when radiotherapy is likely to involve the renal areas.

8.13 Loin pain and haematuria syndrome

A number of patients (predominantly women) have been described who have severe, usually bilateral, loin pain, fever and haematuria. Examination reveals tender loins, with normal blood pressure. Investigation confirms haematuria but no excess proteinuria or infection, normal renal function, and a normal urogram. Renal arteriography shows abnormalities of the intra-renal vascular tree with areas of poor vascularity, and a renal biopsy demonstrates minor abnormalities of the blood vessels.

The cause of the condition is unknown. In some patients there appears to be a relationship with oral contraceptives. Treatment is totally unsatisfactory; the condition responds poorly to analgesics, antibiotics, anticoagulants, antiplatelet agents, steroids and denervation of the kidney.

9: Congenital and inherited renal disease

9.1 Introduction

This chapter is concerned mainly with those conditions likely to be encountered in adults, although some which are often found in children are added for the sake of completeness. The following terms are used in this chapter:

AD: autosomal dominant
AR: autosomal recessive
X-linked: X-linked recessive gene

9.2 Cystic disease of the kidney

Infantile polycystic disease (AR)

This probably consists of more than one variety, depending on the age of onset. The most severe form presents at birth with bilateral renal enlargement, renal failure and associated abnormalities of lung (hypoplasia) and liver (hepatic fibrosis). Other varieties of childhood polycystic diseases present later and have varying degrees of periportal fibrosis. Thus, the younger children tend to die of renal failure and the older children of hepatic failure. There is no known treatment.

Cystic disease of the medulla (AD), juvenile nephronophthisis (AR)

There is disagreement about whether these conditions should be linked together, but they show similar pathological appearances (medullary cysts with cortical interstitial nephritis) and present with polyuria, salt loss and renal failure. Confirmatory tests are difficult since urograms are unhelpful and renal biopsy shows interstitial nephritis. Other abnormalities include retinal and neurological abnormalities. Some patients may present in the second decade with a long history of polyuria and a capacious bladder. There is no known treatment but transplantation has been successfully undertaken.

Adult polycystic disease (AD)

This is a widely distributed familial renal abnormality which accounts for about 10% of adults with renal failure reported in the *European Dialysis and Transplant Registry*. Patients usually present at about the age of 30−40 (rarely younger, occasionally older) with a variety of symptoms including haematuria, hypertension, loin pain, renal failure and urinary tract infection. Abdominal examination shows two large (occasionally massive) kidneys. Confirmation can be undertaken using ultrasound or a CT scan. Cysts may also occur in the liver (commonly) and pancreas (rarely).

Renal failure tends to develop very slowly in patients with polycystic kidneys. Despite hypertension, patients are often sodium losers and require salt supplements, e.g. during operation under a general anaesthetic.

Complications
These include *subarachnoid haemorrhage* due to an increased incidence of berry aneurysms. Haemorrhage may occur before or after starting haemodialysis. Patients who develop a subarachnoid haemorrhage may be switched to peritoneal dialysis or be transplanted in order to avoid heparinization.

Infection may occur in polycystic kidneys often with a *Proteus* or *Pseudomonas* organism. The infection may be difficult to eradicate especially in the presence of renal failure. Treatment with a suitable antibiotic should be continued for 1 month.

Haematuria occurs frequently in patients with polycystic disease. It is often trivial, but in patients on dialysis may be heavy and persistent, necessitating nephrectomy.

Rare complications of polycystic kidneys include renal calcification, tuberculosis, and the development of neoplasms.

Prenatal screening
Patients with polymorphic kidney disease may request genetic counselling. Pregnant women with polycystic kidneys may soon be offered antenatal screening and therapeutic abortion,

since some families with polycystic disease show a mutation on the short arm of chromosome 16. The ethical dilemmas involved are considerable since some patients with polycystic kidneys live normally into their sixties before developing renal failure.

Solitary renal cysts

These are relatively common, especially in older people. Most are asymptomatic, a few patients complain of loin or abdominal fullness or, rarely, develop an upper urinary tract infection. Diagnosis is made by ultrasound and urography. Cyst aspiration may be undertaken either under ultrasound or X-ray screening. Fluid should be sent for microscopy, culture and sensitivity, acid-fast bacilli and cytology. Ultrasound is able to differentiate cysts from solid tumours and arteriography or surgical exploration is rarely necessary.

Calyceal cysts

These are one variety of simple cyst usually revealed by pyelography (see Fig. 8.1). They may be confused with papillary necrosis or tuberculosis. Complications of calyceal cysts include infection, stones and haematuria.

Peripelvic cysts

These are of renal or lymphatic origin and arise in or near the renal hilum. They are usually discovered as an incidental finding on urography and rarely give rise to symptoms.

Medullary sponge kidney

This is diagnosed radiologically when the medulla appears to contain dilated tubules (see Fig. 8.1). The kidney may be larger than normal. Patients present with urinary infections, calculi or haematuria. Some patients have hypercalciuria, most are unable to concentrate the urine. The long-term outlook is excellent.

9.3 Hereditary nephritis

This is probably a heterogenous group of disorders in children presenting with haematuria, proteinuria, deafness and progressive renal failure. They may be divided into hereditary nephritis with deafness (Alport's syndrome) and hereditary nephritis without deafness.

Alport's syndrome
Alport's syndrome is an X-linked abnormality characterized by renal disease (haematuria, proteinuria and an abnormal glomerular basement membrane on electron-microscopy) with high tone sensineural deafness and ophthalmic signs (lenticoma and macular flecks). Boys tend to be more severely affected than girls with renal failure appearing earlier and a high incidence of deafness and eye changes. Gene linkage studies have suggested the locus responsible for this disease is situated in the region Yq 11−22 on the long arm of the X-chromosome. Affected male patients as well as apparently non-affected female relatives may require genetic counselling.

Hereditary nephritis without deafness
There are undoubtedly other patients who have renal abnormalities similar to classical Alport's syndrome, but who do not develop deafness. Families may show great variability in the seriousness of their renal disease. The genetics of these disorders is under discussion but may involve an autosomal dominant gene or less likely, an autorecessive state.

9.4 Renal tubular defects

A number of renal defects in the handling of various substances have been described. Most are rare, some extremely so; the more common forms are shown in the Table 9.1.

In addition to various tubular abnormalities there are a large number of dysplastic, cystic and inflammatory renal lesions that are associated with an astonishing variety of disorders of the ears, eyes, skeleton, viscera, chromosomal and metabolic abnormalities. A review of the principle varieties,

Table 9.1 Renal tubular handling defects.

Handling defect	Biochemical findings and clinical features	Genetics	Treatment
Renal glycosuria	Glycosuria. None	X-linked	None
Amino-aciduria			
Glycinuria	Mainly normal	AR	None needed
Cystinuria (see p. 177)	Cystine, ornithine, lysine arginine in urine. Cystine stones	AR	(see p. 177)
Hartnup disease	Multiple amino acid abnormalities. Pellagra, cerebellar ataxia, delirium	AR	Nicotinamide
Hypophosphataemia	Hypophosphataemia and phosphaturia. Rickets	X-linked	Vitamin D and oral phosphate
Renal tubular acidosis	Hyperchloraemic compensated acidosis with low bicarbonate	AD	See p. 36

	Features	Inheritance	Treatment
Lowe's syndrome	Amino-aciduria, hypophosphataemia and tubular acidosis. Cataracts, glaucoma, mental retardation and failure to thrive	X-linked or AR	Bicarbonate, vitamin D
Nephrogenic diabetes insipidus	Failure to thrive, hyposthenuria, hypernatraemia, fever, vomiting, constipation	Variable	Water, thiazide diuretics
Adult Fanconi's syndrome*	Renal glycosuria, amino-aciduria, phosphaturia and renal tubular acidosis. Rickets or osteomalacia, rarely renal failure	AR	Treat underlying metabolic defects
Lignac—Fanconi syndrome (cystinosis, cystine storage disease)	Deposits of cystine crystals in tissues, amino-aciduria, glycosuria, phosphaturia. Failure to thrive, hypokalaemia, proteinuria, rickets, renal failure	AR	Dialysis, transplantation

* Note that adult Fanconi's syndrome may be secondary to poisoning with heavy metals, amyloidosis, sickle-cell disease, or other inborn errors of metabolism (e.g. Wilson's disease).

renal abnormalities and inheritance is given by Chantler in an appendix in Rubin and Barratt (eds) (*Paediatric Nephrology* 1975, Williams and Wilkins, Baltimore).

9.5 HLA system and renal disease

It is becoming increasingly apparent that some forms of glomerulonephritis and arteritis are associated with certain HLA genotypes. The reasons for this are not entirely clear but relate perhaps to the close proximity of the HLA determinants to various complement components on the short arm of chromosome 6 (Fig. 9.1).

The conditions linked to certain HLA types are shown in Table 9.2.

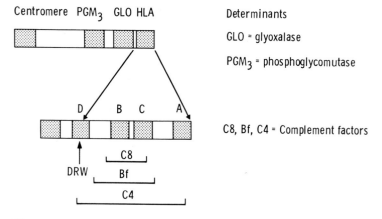

Fig. 9.1 Regions on the short arm of chromosome 6.

Table 9.2 Conditions linked to HLA types.

Condition	HLA type
Minimal change GN	B12 DR7 DRW7
Membranous GN	B8 B18 DRW3
Goodpasture's disease	B7 DR2 DR3
Mesangial IgA GN	BW35 — possibly associated with deteriorating renal function

9.6 Other renal diseases and familial tendencies

Reflux nephropathy
This condition is occasionally familial: some authors have stressed the importance of family screening.

Familial Mediterranean fever (AR)
This presents in childhood with joint pain (serositis) and synovitis (but no joint malformation), fever and a tendency to develop amyloidosis. Symptomatic treatment for the joint pain is required together with colchicine for fever. Long-term colchicine may also prevent or arrest amyloid formation.

Fabry's disease
Fabry's disease is an X-linked recessive disorder resulting in painful extremities, angiokeratomas, telangiectasases with proteinuria, and renal failure. Renal biopsy shows a characteristic 'myelin' figure on electron microscopy. There is no known treatment.

Tuberous sclerosis
Tuberous sclerosis is an autosomal dominant disorder with a high mutation rate affecting chromosome 9. The disease results in adenoma sebaceans, mental retardation, epilepsy, renal angiolipomata and eventually renal failure.

10: Renal stone disease

10.1 Introduction

Renal stone disease is of importance to general physicians and nephro-urologists alike. The principle kinds of renal stones and their main characteristics are set out in Table 10.1.

Investigation

Investigation of patients with renal calculi include the following.
1 Stone analysis, wherever possible.
2 Blood tests: FBC, ESR; tests for urea, sodium, potassium, chloride, bicarbonate, creatinine, creatinine clearance, uric acid (twice), calcium and phosphate (three times), alkaline phosphatase, serum proteins, PTH.
3 Urine tests: a 24 hour collection of calcium oxalate and urate (twice); random urine pH, cystine screen; MSU microscopy, culture and sensitivity; early morning urine (EMU) for tuberculous bacilli.
4 Radiology: plain film, urography, hand X-rays.

Special investigations
- ammonium chloride test to exclude renal tubular acidosis
- phosphate threshold (see Appendix 2)
- serum ionized calcium

10.2 Primary hyperparathyroidism

This is a relatively rare cause of renal stones representing $5-10\%$ of all patients with stones. The characteristics of renal stones can be seen on Table 10.1. Approximately $50-60\%$ of patients with hyperparathyroidism develop stones. The metabolic discrimination between stone-formers and non-stone-formers may be due to higher levels of serum $1-25$ vitamin D_3 in stone-formers, resulting in greater calcium absorption.

Table 10.1 Characteristics of various renal stones.

Type of stone	Approximate occurrence (%)	Main causes	X-ray appearances	Solubility
Calcium } oxalate Magnesium } phosphate	70	Hyperparathyroidism, hypercalciuria, hyperuricosuria, high urine pH, none of these	Opaque	Increased in acid urine
Calcium Magnesium } phosphate Ammonium	20	Infection	Opaque	
Urate	5	Gout, hyperuricosuria	Translucent	Increased in alkaline urine
Cystine	4	Cystinuria		

Patients with hyperparathyroidism have:
- hypercalcaemia (this may be borderline and two or three estimations may be required)
- hypophosphataemia
- low serum bicarbonate with type two renal tubular acidosis
- hypercalciuria, hyperphosphaturia
- raised ionized calcium, raised PTH

Borderline cases (minor elevation of serum calcium, low serum phosphate with hypercalciuria) may pose special problems in diagnosis and the use of the phosphate threshold test (see Appendix 2) may help to distinguish hyperparathyroidism from other causes of hypercalciuria.

Treatment
This is by exploration of the neck with removal of an adenoma or subtotal parathyroidectomy if there is parathyroid hyperplasia.

10.3 Idiopathic hypercalciuria

In this condition the 24-hour urine calcium level is >7.5 mmol (300 mg) in men and >6.1 mmol (250 mg) in women. These high levels may be due to:
- a high intake of calcium
- absorbtive hypercalciuria (partially due to increased $1-25$ OH vitamin D_3 production)
- renal calcium leak

Some investigators put patients with hypercalciuria on a low (<6.1 mmol) calcium diet for 3 days to exclude hyperabsorption of calcium as a likely cause of hypercalciuria.

Treatment

Treatment is directed towards reducing calcium excretion. The following measures have been tried.

Thiazide diuretics
Administration of, for example, bendrofluazide 5 mg daily, reduces calcium excretion by increasing calcium resorption in

the distal tubule. Side-effects are uncommon but periodic checks of potassium, urate and glucose levels are required.

Cellulose phosphate
15 g daily acts by binding gut calcium but may aggravate secondary hyperparathyroidism and increase urinary oxalate excretion.

Diet and fluid intake
A low calcium diet helps to reduce urinary calcium excretion and patients with idiopathic hypercalciuria should avoid dairy products. Increasing fluid intake is also recommended but difficult to sustain. To be effective, a patient should pass urine at least once during the night. Certain liquids, e.g. hard water, may contribute to the dietary calcium load and drinks rich in oxalate, e.g. tea, are also to be avoided.

10.4 Calcium oxalate stones with hyperuricosuria

This is becoming increasingly recognized as an important cause of stone formation. The urinary uric acid level is > 4.4 mmol (800 mg) in men and > 3.8 mmol (700 mg) in women. By definition these patients do not have hypercalcaemia, gout or hyperoxaluria. Hypercalciuria or slight rises in serum urate may be present. Calcium oxalate stones form either by crystals of sodium urate acting as a nucleus for calcium oxalate, or uric acid (as urate crystals) absorbing inhibitors of crystal growth.

Treatment
- reduce dietary protein and purine intake
- give allopurinol 300 mg daily

10.5 Hyperoxaluria

Oxalate is difficult to measure, but ranges from 15–50 mg per 24 hours with a mean of 35 mg. Most renal stones contain oxalate, but most stone-formers do not excrete excess oxalate. Oxalate is widely distributed in foods (see Appendix 6). Its absorption is determined, in part, by dietary calcium content, since a low dietary calcium enhances oxalate absorption. The main causes of hyperoxaluria are:

- gastro-intestinal disorders (enteric hyperoxaluria)
- increased oxalate intake
- primary hyperoxaluria
- increased intake of oxalate precusors
- pyridoxine deficiency

Enteric

A number of different bowel disorders, including Crohn's disease, malabsorption (blind loops, bacterial overgrowth, non-tropical sprue, pancreatitis) and surgical resection or bypass of the small bowel have been associated with the development of oxalate stones. Various aetiologies have been proposed, including the presence of bile acids in the colon which increase the absorption of oxalate and complex calcium which is then unavailable to bind oxalate. Patients with diarrhoea have lower urine outputs resulting in concentrated urine. Moreover, bicarbonate, is lost in the faeces, the urine remains acid, and citrate excretion is reduced, allowing crystal growth of both calcium phosphate and calcium oxalate.

Patients present with renal colic, renal failure, or the stones may be discovered accidentally on X-ray. Treatment consists of:

- calcium carbonate (precipitates oxalate in the bowels)
- increasing fluid intake
- avoiding foods high in oxalate (see Appendix 6)
- specific treatment for the underlying bowel disorder, a low fat diet, cholestyramine, alkali replacement if metabolic acidosis is present, magnesium replacement for magnesium deficiency, and allopurinol if concurrent uric acid stones are present

Primary

This is a very rare disorder of oxalate metabolism consisting of two types (I and II), each with distinct enzyme deficiencies.

The disease starts in early childhood and is associated with a high morbidity and mortality. Death results from renal failure and oxalosis. Treatment consists of pyridoxine, orthophosphates and magnesium or phosphate supplements.

Other rare causes

Excess intake of ascorbic acid (>4 g per day), ethylene glycol intoxication, methoxyflurane anaesthesia, infection with aspergillosis and pyridoxine deficiency, have all been described as causing hyperoxaluria and oxalate stones.

10.6 Calcium stones of undetermined origin
(excluding hyperparathyroidism, hypercalciuria, and hyperoxaluria)

The aetiology of the stones in this group of stone-formers is speculative but includes increased urinary calcium concentration (decreased urine volume), abnormal handling of calcium by the kidney (increased distal tubule calcium concentration), increased phosphate, oxalate and urate concentration, and a reduction in urinary inhibitors. Methods of treatment are shown in Table 10.2.

Reduced dietary protein and purine, plus high fluid intake should be the first step. Use thiazide and allopurinol with low oxalate diet if the stones recur. If thiazide diuretics or allopurinol are not tolerated, use orthophosphates, with magnesium salts and/or pyridoxine.

10.7 Uric acid stones

Uric acid deposition in the kidney may occur as:
- interstitial deposition of monosodium urate in patients with gout
- acute deposition of uric acid in patients with lymphoproliferative and myeloproliferative diseases
- formation of uric acid calculi

The following conditions are associated with the development of uric acid stones:

Table 10.2 Methods of treatment for calcium stones of undetermined origin.

Method	Notes
High fluid intake	Beware hard water (install water softener?)
Low calcium diet ⎱ Low oxalate diet ⎰	Little effect if dietary calcium is already normal. This treatment may potentiate hyperoxaluria, therefore oxalate content should be reduced as well
Low sodium diet Low purine diet Reduced protein intake	All may work; no controlled studies are available. A high protein, high purine diet is to be avoided
Thiazide diuretics	These have been shown to be effective. They reduce urinary oxalate and may increase urinary magnesium
Inorganic phosphate	Some evidence suggests that orthophosphate may be effective. Diarrhoea is likely if > 2 g per day is taken. Other effects include a transient increase in parathyroid hormone
Cellulose phosphate	Use only if there is hyperabsorption of calcium
Allopurinol (300 mg per day) Magnesium salts Pyridoxine	These may be helpful, especially if used with thiazides. All have been used singly and in combination. Magnesium salts induce diarrhoea

- primary gout
- myeloproliferative disorder
- administration of uricosuric drugs
- inherited enzyme deficiencies, e.g. hypoxanthine guanine phosphoribosyl transferase (HGPT) deficiency, or G6PD deficiency
- high protein diet
- alcohol
- low urine pH

Uric acid stones may be radio-translucent. Diagnosis is confirmed by stone analysis.

Treatment

The treatment of any underlying disorder, obesity, alcoholism, and excess purine intake, is first required. Unfortunately, many patients find adherence to a strict diet difficult, and patients with genetic abnormalities will have hyperuricosuria despite dietary manipulation. For most patients allopurinol, (300 mg daily with normal renal function) and, possibly, urinary alkalinization and increased fluid intake, will be required.

10.8 Cystinuria

This is an autosomal recessive abnormality of proximal tubular and intestinal transport of cystine, ornithine, lysine and arginine (COLA or COAL). In the major variety of cystinuria, active intestinal transport of cystine, arginine and lysine is absent, and the urinary excretion of all four amino acids is increased. There are various subsets of the disease based on differences in intestinal transport, but all homozygotes have an increased urinary amino acid excretion. Malnutrition is prevented by the absorption of peptides. Cystine stones form because cystine is the least soluble of the four amino acids.

Cystinuria is a rare cause of partially radio-translucent calculi (cystine stones are slightly more radio-opaque than urate stones). Diagnosis is made by examining urine for 'benzene ring' crystals, (p. 25), screening by means of the cyanide-nitroprusside test, and ultimately by amino acid analysis of the patient's urine when the excretion of the relevant amino acids may be up to five times the normal.

Treatment

1 Adequate fluid intake up to 3–4 litres per day. It can be calculated that, as cystine precipitates more than 300 mg/l of urine, (at a pH of 4.5–7.0) the total amount of urine to be passed is 3.3 multiplied by x where x is the cystine excretion (in mg) per 24 hours.

2 Alkalinization is not really effective until the urine pH is about 7.5, requiring 5–10 g of sodium bicarbonate per day. One possible complication is calcium phosphate precipitation.

3 D-Penicillamine combines with cystine to form a soluble complex (cysteine-disulphide). In adults, 1–2 g of penicillamine will reduce free urinary cystine to 100–150 mg per day. Unfortunately, penicillamine has a high incidence of side-effects, including rashes, blood dyscrasias, loss of taste, proteinuria, SLE reaction, pemphigus, poor collagen production, and gastrointestinal intolerance.

10.9 Infection-associated stones

All renal stones may be complicated by infection but one particular variety of stone (struvite or calcium, magnesium, ammonium phosphate) is associated with urea-splitting organisms (urease producers, notably *Proteus* spp.).

Most stones of this type present as staghorn calculi with episodes of upper urinary infection, odour to the urine, haematuria or renal colic. Patients with some underlying radiological renal damage are likely to develop calculus if disease infection occurs with urease-producing organisms.

Treatment
Antimicrobial therapy suppresses rather than eradicates infection. However, long-term treatment with antibiotics such as co-trimoxazole, ampicillin or a cephalosporin, may reduce bacterial numbers sufficiently to prevent new stone formation.

Surgery remains the most important part in the management of patients with infection-induced stones.

A novel approach has been to use certain compounds, e.g. hydroxyurea or acetohydroxamic acid (AHA) to inhibit urease, thereby blocking new stone formation. Unfortunately, both compounds are toxic and not available for the treatment of infection stones.

Nephrocalcinosis
Nephrocalcinosis may be due to:
- renal tubular acidosis
- medullary sponge kidney
- sarcoidosis
- calcified papillae
- hyperparathyroidism (rare)

Surgical management of stones
Details of this topic are outside the scope of this text but the
last few years have seen a revolution in the surgical management of calculi with the introduction of percutaneous stone
removal and the use of the lithotripter.

11: Hypertension and the kidney

11.1 Factors determining blood pressure in patients with renal disease

The blood pressure is determined by the cardiac output and peripheral resistance. High blood pressure results from either an increase in output or peripheral resistance or both. A summary of various factors and their inter-relationships is given in Fig. 11.1.

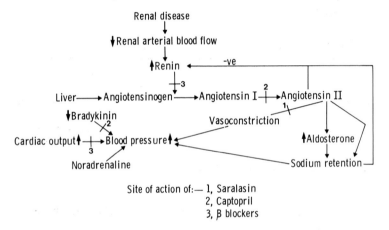

Fig. 11.1 Factors and their inter-relationships which determine blood pressure in patients with renal disease.

The concept of a dual regulation of blood pressure mediated by angiotensin II and sodium retention has been verified both experimentally and in clinical practice. Changes in cardiac output govern the results of treatment rather than act as an aetiological factor. As sodium retention inhibits the release of renin, patients are divided into either 'volume-dependent' or 'renin-dependent' groups, but this notion does not take into account other vasoconstrictor or vasodilator factors, e.g. autonomic dysfunction, noradrenaline or bradykinin. Furthermore, in any one patient both volume and angiotensin control are mixed.

11.2 Investigation of high blood pressure

There is considerable debate about the levels at which 'hypertension' should be investigated, and what investigation should be undertaken. In general, a consistent (taken two or three times over an interval of one week) blood pressure of > 150/100 mmHg in patients under the age of 40 and > 160/100 mmHg over that age, should be investigated and treated.

Hypertension may result from any of the conditions shown in Table 11.1.

Table 11.1 Various conditions which can result in hypertension.

Renal	Non-renal
Major renal vascular disease	Coarctation of the aorta
Any renal pathological abnormality, unilateral or bilateral	Endocrine causes:
	phaeochromocytoma
	primary aldosterone
	Cushing's disease

The following investigations may be undertaken in a patient with hypertension.

Haematology: routine blood tests — FBC, ESR.

Biochemistry: urea, electrolytes, creatinine, creatinine clearance, and vanilmandelic acid (VMA) excretion tests, lipids and glucose. In selected patients only, protein excretion, plasma renin activity (PRA) and aldosterone levels.

Bacteriology: MSU, for microscopy culture and sensitivity.

Radiology: plain X-ray of the abdomen, CXR, urogram, and in selected patients only, arteriogram.

Other: ECG.

11.3 Renal hypertension

Renal artery stenosis

This is a rare cause of hypertension. It is due either to fibro-muscular hyperplasia in patients (usually women under the age of 40) or atheroma (mainly in patients over the age of 40). The diagnosis is confirmed by:
• IVU: the affected side is smaller (by at least 2 cm), has delayed concentration and delay in filling the ureter; rarely, there is ureteral notching
• renogram shows delay in peak of normal outflow
• arteriogram shows stenotic lesion with post-stenotic dilatation

The problem arises as to whether the anatomical abnormality is matched by a corresponding functional abnormality likely to be reversed by surgery. Several tests have been described, including measurement of renal vein renin, when several samples should be obtained from both renal veins and compared to the peripheral vein renin. A ratio of greater than 1.5 : 1 or 2.0 : 1 comparing the PRA from the affected side to the peripheral venous concentration, has been considered as an indication of a likely favourable response to surgery. If the non-stenotic renal venous renin concentration is also high then the outlook for surgery is poor, due to established renal vascular disease in the non-stenotic kidney.

The administration of captopril (an angiotensin converting enzyme inhibitor) reduces renal blood flow in kidneys whose blood supply is reduced in renal artery stenosis, combined with renography is under evaluation.

The choice of whether to operate on any particular patient depends on the age, nature of stenosis and history of previous vascular disease. Patients over the age of 50 with atheromatous lesions, and a previous history of vascular disease, do not respond to surgery as well as patients below the age of 40 with fibromuscular hyperplasia and no other vascular lesion.

There is an increasing tendency to treat renal arterial stenosis whether or not associated with a functional abnormality especially as the presence of renal failure. Angioplasty, although preferable technically to arterial repair, may have a higher rate of restenosis. Bilateral renal artery stenosis is an important cause of renal failure in the elderly.

Other causes

Other causes should become apparent as soon as various investigations of renal structure and function are known. Unilateral renal diseases other than renal artery stenosis that are likely to cause hypertension are reflux nephropathy or, rarely, obstruction. Neither of these conditions is likely to respond to nephrectomy since the abnormality has usually been present for years and damage to the contralateral kidney has occurred.

11.4 Non-renal causes of hypertension

1 *Coarctation* of the aorta is rare but should be excluded by careful physical examination comparing arm to leg pulses.

Phaeochromocytoma
2 *Phaeochromocytoma* should be suspected if a patient with hypertension also complains of sweating, palpitations and headaches.

Diagnostic tests for phaeochromocytoma are shown in Table 11.2. In borderline cases suppression or stimulation tests may be used.

Table 11.2 Diagnostic tests for phaeochromocytoma.

Test	Normal range	Sensitivity	Specificity
Urinary VMA	< 40 μmol (8 mg)/24 hours	0.42	1.00
Urinary catecholamine	< 9.5 μmol (1.8 mg)/ 24 hours	0.79	0.93
Plasma catecholamine	< 5.62 nmol/l (950 pg/ml)	0.94	0.97

Modified from Bravo EL and Gifford RW, (1984) *New Eng J Med* **311**: 1298–1303.

Suppression tests
Oral clonidine 0.3 mg followed by plasma catecholamines hourly for 3 hours.
Result: plasma catecholamine less than 500 pg/ml in essential hypertension.

Stimulation tests
Glucagon 1.0−2.0 mg i.v.
Result: increase in plasma catecholamines above 2000 pg/ml or threefold increase 1−3 minutes after administration. Increase in BP of at least 20/15 above cold pressor test (not essential).

Localization of tumour
- CAT scan
- MIBG scans using iodinated cholesterol

Management
β-blocking drugs should not be given alone to patients with phaeochromocytomas for fear of promoting a hypertension crisis. α-blocking drugs (e.g. phenoxybenzamine) should be included pre- and during any operations to prevent swings of blood pressure. Labetalol, an α- and β-blocking drug, has been used successfully in the pre-operative management of patients with phaeochromocytomas.

3 Primary aldosteronism (see below).
4 Cushings' disease.

Hypertension and hypokalaemia

This is an important association requiring an explanation in any individual case. Likely causes include:
- treatment with diuretics
- primary aldosteronism, Cushing's syndrome
- secondary aldosteronism
- potassium loss of some other cause in a patient with essential hypertension.
- renin-secreting tumours

The diagnosis can usually be differentiated by measurement of renin and aldosterone after a period of withdrawal of all hypotensives and simultaneous measurements of urinary sodium excretion. Various findings are set out in Table 11.3.

Table 11.3 Differential diagnosis of 1° and 2° hyperaldosteronism.

	Primary aldosteronism	Secondary aldosteronism*
Plasma sodium	↑	↔
Plasma potassium	↓	↓
Plasma renin	↓	↑
Aldosterone	↑	↑
Extracellular fluid volume	Variable	Variable

↑ : Increased, ↔: normal, ↓ : reduced.
* e.g. accelerated hypertension, chronic renal disease, renal artery stenosis, or renin-secreting tumour.

5 *Renin-secreting tumours* are an extremely rare cause of hypertension occurring in young people who have hypertension, hypokalaemia, raised aldosterone secretion, raised plasma renin activity and a normal renal vascular tree. Small intra-renal tumours may be found which secrete renin.

11.5 Essential hypertension

By definition, this is a high blood pressure of unknown cause, e.g. when all screening tests for renal or endocrine causes are negative. There does not seem, at present, any indication for routine screening of patients with aldosterone or renin levels.

11.6 Malignant hypertension (some prefer the term 'accelerated' hypertension)

Almost any form of hypertension may present as either benign or malignant (accelerated) hypertension. Malignant hypertension (papilloedema, haemorrhages and exudates) has a poor prognosis from progressive renal failure, cerebrovascular accidents and other vascular problems.

11.7 Treatment of hypertension

There is debate as to what level and at what age high blood pressure should be treated. Most physicians agree that pressures of > 180 mmHg systolic and > 110 mmHg diastolic should be treated, irrespective of age. Lesser degrees of hypertension, e.g. 150/100 mmHg in patients of 65 years may not require treatment but at the age of 40 should be treated.

Mild hypertension (BP 150−170/100−110)

Most patients with mild hypertension will respond to salt restriction and weight reduction if obese. The relative merits of thiazide diuretics, β-blockers and calcium channel blockers is debatable. Simple dose regimens will ensure compliance.

Moderate to severe hypertension (BP 170−190/110−120)

This usually requires treatment with drugs such as calcium channel blockers, β-blockers, vasodilators, diuretics or ACE inhibitors alone or in combination, e.g.:
- β-blockers + calcium channel blockers
- β-blockers + hydralazine
- β-blockers + diuretics

Considerable controversy surrounds which drug or groups of drugs to use. Once daily administration will secure compliance.

Accelerated (malignant) hypertension

Angiotensin-converting enzyme inhibitors such as captopril or enalapril may be used with caution but are theoretically the drugs of choice since angiotensin levels are high. The drugs should be given in very small doses (e.g. captopril 6.25 mg as a starting dose) and the blood pressure measured at 15 minute intervals. Patients with accelerated hypertension and renal failure may show further reduction in renal function which should be monitored with great care. Parenteral therapy is rarely required but the following drugs have been used:
- hydralazine 10−20 mg i.m.
- labetalol 50 mg i.v.
- sodium nitroprusside (0.5−1.5 µg/kg i.v with a maximum dose of 80 µg per minute)

Indications and contraindications for individual hypotensive agents are shown in Table 11.4.

Table 11.4 Indications and contraindications for hypotensive agents.

Drug	Indications	Contraindication
Thiazide diuretic	Elderly patient Volume dependent, e.g. steroid-induced, black patients	Diabetes Gout Marked hyperlipidaemia
β-blockers	Young hypertensives History of myocardial infarction History of angina Mitral valve prolapse	Obstructive airways disease Peripheral vascular disease Diabetes
Calcium channel blockers	Elderly hypertensives Black hypertensives Hypertension and peripheral vascular disease Hypertension and obstructive airways disease	History of migraine
ACE inhibitor	Malignant hypertension Hypertension and diabetes Hypertension and renal failure Hypertension and cardiac failure	Tendency to hyperkalaemia

11.8 Pregnancy and high blood pressure

Definitions of pre-eclampsia vary but all include hypertension
(> 140/90 mmHg on two occasions 24 hours apart, or a rise
of > 30 mmHg systolic or 15 mmHg diastolic pressure
from pre-pregnancy or early pregnancy levels). Proteinuria
(> 0.5 g per 24 hours) is an optional extra in the definition;
oedema occurs so often in pregnancy that it should no longer
be included. The cause of pre-eclampsia is unknown and probably multifactorial. Assessment and treatment of hypertension
in pregnancy is important, for the risks to both mother and
fetus are high. Important steps in management include:
• exclusion of other causes of hypertension (phaeochromocytoma, coarctation, renal diseases)
• assessment of maternal renal function (urea, creatinine
clearance, urate, MSU)
• assessment of fetal well-being

Treatment

Mild pre-eclampsia (BP (140−160)/(90−100) mmHg) may be
managed by rest and careful observation. There is no need to
treat these patients with hypotensive drugs or diuretics. Most
obstetricians would induce labour at 38 weeks.

Severe pre-eclampsia

(BP > 160/> 100 mmHg, usually with proteinuria) requires
admission to hospital and careful maternal and fetal monitoring. If hyperreflexia or fits occur, diazepam (2−4 mg per hour)
or magnesium sulphate (4−6 g i.v. at 1 g per hour, providing
renal function is normal) are given. Hypertension may be
treated with hydralazine (10 mg t.d.s.) and methyldopa may
be added. In most cases, the fetus should be delivered by
caesarean section, and sedatives should continue for 48 hours
after delivery. Disseminated intravascular coagulation can
occur at any time and relevant tests should be part of maternal
monitoring.

Table 11.5 Investigation of disorders of the renin–angiotensin system.

Disorder	Plasma Na⁺	Plasma K⁺	Urinary Na⁺	Urinary K⁺	Renin	Aldosterone	BP	ECF
Barrter's syndrome	N	↓	V	↑	↑	↑	N	N
Surreptitious vomiting	V	↓	↓	↑	↑	↑	↓	↓
Diuretic abuse	V	↓	↑	↑	↑	↑	V	↓
Liquorice abuse	↑	↓	↓	↑	↓	↓	↑	↑
Laxative abuse	V	↓	↓	↑	↑	↑	↓	↓
Hyporeninaemic hypoaldosteronism	↓	↑	↑	↓	↓	↓	↓	↓
Adrenal insufficiency	↓	↑	↑	↓	↑	↓	↓	↓
Primary aldosteronism	↑	↓	V	↑	↓	↑	↑	↑
Renovascular disease	N	V	V	V	↑	↑	↑	N

N: normal;   V: variable;   ↑ : increased;   ↓ : decreased

Post-delivery assessment

By 6 weeks post-partum, the blood pressure of patients with pregnancy-induced hypertension should have returned to normal. If hypertension or proteinuria persist, relevant investigation as for any non-pregnant patient should be undertaken.

Pregnancy in pre-existing renal disease and patients with essential hypertension

If patients present with hypertension within the first trimester, renal function tests and a search for any likely cause of hypertension must be undertaken. The general principles for the management of pregnancy-induced hypertension apply. Certain hypotensive drugs (β-blockers, diuretics, ganglion-blocking drugs, diazoxide and ACE inhibitors) are to be avoided, leaving methyldopa with or without hydralazine as the drug of choice.

Patients with renal failure are less likely to conceive, but adequate contraception should be practised if unwanted pregnancies are to be avoided. The effect of a pregnancy on underlying renal disease is controversial; in some groups (e.g. reflux nephropathy) renal function may worsen.

11.9 Disorders of the renin–angiotensin–aldosterone system

Disorders associated with hypertension are discussed on p. 184. Those associated with normal blood pressure include a variety of interesting and fairly rare problems, many of which present with hypokalaemia.

Barrter's syndrome is characterized by hypokalaemia, hypochloraemia, alkalosis, hyper-reninism, hyperaldosteronism, normotension and resistance to the pressor effect of exogenous angiotensin II. Hyperplasia of the renal juxta glomerular apparatus is seen. Most cases occur in childhood and there is a familial tendency. The precise cause is uncertain but a defect in tubular sodium or chloride transport has been suggested. One striking feature is that most of the defects of Barrter's syndrome can be reversed by prostaglandin inhibitors (e.g.

indomethacin) but it is unclear whether the excess renal prostaglandin production is a primary or secondary effect.

Other disorders of the renin-angiotensin system, and the relevant investigations, are given in Table 11.5.

12: Drugs and the kidney

12.1 The kidney and drug overdoses

Alteration of urinary pH to speed drug elimination is shown in Table 12.1.

Table 12.1 Alteration of urinary pH to speed drug elimination.

Alkaline urine	Acid urine
Phenobarbitone	Pethidine
Aspirin	Morphine
	Amphetamines
	Fenfluramine

In practice, alkalinization is useful for the elimination of phenobarbitone and aspirin when aspirin levels are between 500 and 800 mg/l (if > 800 mg/l use haemodialysis) and when phenobarbitone levels are between 50 and 100 mg/l (if > 100 mg/l use haemodialysis). Alkalinization is achieved by administration of sodium bicarbonate, and the urine pH should be greater than 7. The serum potassium level should be checked 6 hourly, and the calcium level daily. Aspirin overdosage induces complex metabolic problems and serum pH, P_{CO_2} and P_{O_2} must be monitored.

Urinary acidification is more difficult to achieve. Ammonium chloride causes nausea, and cannot be given intravenously. Arginine or lysine hydrochloride have been given. In practice, opiate overdosage is best treated by naloxone, and amphetamine overdosage by sedation with chlorpromazine or a short-acting barbiturate.

Poisons and haemodialysis

There are a limited number of substances that can be removed by haemodialysis, including those shown in Table 12.2.

Table 12.2 Substances that can be removed by haemodialysis.

Drugs	Poisons
Lithium	Methyl alcohol
* Phenobarbitone	Ethyl alcohol
* Salicylates	Ethylene glycol

* These may be preferentially treated by
forced alkaline diuresis

Haemoperfusion

Haemoperfusion has been used to reduce the blood concentration of a number of drugs but should be reserved for severe clinical intoxication including coma, hypotension, hypothermia, progressive clinical deterioration, and high blood levels of the following drugs:

- phenobarbitone > 100 mg/l
- salicylates > 800 mg/l

May be preferentially treated by haemodialysis or forced alkaline diuresis

- barbitone > 100 mg/l
- other barbiturates > 50 mg/l
- glutethimide > 40 mg/l
- ethchlorvynol > 150 mg/l
- meprobamate > 100 mg/l
- trichlorethanol derivatives > 50 mg/l
- theophylline > 60 mg/l
- paraquat
- mushroom poisoning

Haemodialysis is of no value

Haemoperfusion requires access to the circulation (shunt, subclavian or femoral vein catheter), and facilities for maintaining an extra-corporeal circulation and a perfusion column. Complications include leucopenia and thrombocytopenia and all the complications of an extra-corporeal circuit.

12.2 Drugs causing renal disease

Acute tubular necrosis

Aminoglycosides
- gentamycin ⎫
- tobramycin ⎬ especially with frusemide
- amikacin ⎭

Cephalosporins
- cephalothin ⎫
- cephaloridine ⎬ with or without frusemide

Other antimicrobials
- Colomycin

Poisons
- carbon tetrachloride
- mercuric chloride
- paraquat
- ethylene glycol

Acute interstitial nephritis

- penicillins:
  methicillin
  ampicillin
- sulphonamides including
co-trimoxazole
- cephalosporins
- rifampicin
- phenindione
- phenylbutazone ⎫
- frusemide ⎪
- thiazide diuretics ⎬ rare
- sulphinpyrazone ⎭

Chronic interstitial nephritis

- phenacetin

Exacerbating pre-existing renal failure

- tetracycline (except Doxycyline)
- steroids
- NSAIDS

Distal tubular poisons

- lithium
- anti-leukaemic and neoplastic drugs (via hyperuricaemia)

Retroperitoneal fibrosis

- methysergide
- amphetamines
- phenacetin

- methyldopa
- practalol

SLE-inducing drugs

- hydralazine (> 200 mg/day)
- INAH (iso-nicotinic acid hydrazine)
- procainamide

Bladder irritation

- cyclophosphamide

12.3 Use of drugs in patients with renal failure

A full description of dosage requirements is given in the British National Formulary (*Prescribing in Renal Impairment*). The following points are worth emphasizing in patients on maintenance haemodialysis.

1 Nephrotoxicity is obviously irrelevant in dialysis patients.

2 A large number of drugs are dialysable. It is virtually impossible to maintain accurate levels during dialysis and an extra dose of drug is required at the end of dialysis.

3 There is a tendency for patients on dialysis to be prescribed multiple drugs. This tendency should be resisted!

Remember! Any new drug: How is it excreted? What is the toxicity? Table 12.3 gives a personal selection of drugs to be used in patients on haemodialysis in the stated situation. It is better to be familiar with a limited range of drugs.

Table 12.3 Drugs for use in renal failure.

Indication	Drugs (in order of preference)	Notes
Antacid	Aludrox 10–20 ml q.d.s Ranitidine 150 mg o.d.	Constipates, aluminium toxicity Short-term use only
Antinausea	Metoclopramide 5–10 mg 6 hourly	Extra-pyramidal effects
Antidiarrhoeal	Codeine phosphate 15 mg 4–6 hourly Loperamide 2 mg t.d.s.	Drowsiness may occur
Antipruritus	Emulsifying cream Chlorpheniramine 4 mg 6 hourly Clemastine 1 mg b.d. Ultraviolet light	Usual antihistamine side-effects Check phosphate levels
Analgesic	Paracetamol 0.5–1.0 g 4–6 hourly Cosalgesic i–ii 4–6 hourly	Risk of overdose *Beware opiates* for dialysis patients
Hypnotic	Temazepam 10–20 mg Diazepam 5 mg	Short half-life Morning drowsiness
Anti-inflammatory agents	Paracetamol 0.5–1.0 g 4–6 hourly Indomethacin 25 mg 6 hourly Indomethacin suppositories	Gastro-intestinal bleeding

Hypotensive drugs	Metoprolol	Start with 50 mg b.d.
	Atenalol	Start with 50 mg o.d.
	Hydralazine t.d.s.	No more than 50 mg t.d.s.
	Nifedipine S.R.	10–20 mg b.d.
	Enalapril	5 mg daily
Arrhythmias	Propranolol and other β-blockers	*Avoid* digitalis
	Disopyramide—100 mg daily	
Infections		
Simple shunt infections (identify organism)	Fluscloxacillin 250 mg t.d.s or cephalexin 500 mg daily	Some accumulation possible but blood levels guaranteed
Severe shunt infection (identify organism)	Fluscloxacillin 250 mg t.d.s or cephalexin 500 mg daily, plus tobramycin 1 mg/kg body weight i.m. at end of dialysis	Do not give tobramycin i.v.; inject into thigh, not buttock
Staphylococcal infection including septicaemia	Fluscloxacillin plus tobramycin or vancomycin 1 g i.v. at end of dialysis, diluted in 200 ml NS alone, given over 2 hours *every 7–10 days*	Ease of administration
Suspected septicaemia	Benzyl penicillin 1 g 6–8 hourly Tobramycin loading dose + 1 mg/kg body weight at end of dialysis, with or without metronidazole (if anaerobic) 400 mg t.d.s.	*May* be replaced by newer broad spectrum penicillins or cephalosporins
Urinary tract infections (surprisingly rare)	Cephalexin 500 mg o.d. Co-trimoxazole 1 o.d. Doxycyline 100 mg o.d.	Useful for prostatic infection *Do not* use nitrofurantoin or nalidixic acid

Table 12.3 cont'd

Indication	Drugs (in order of preference)	Notes
Chest infection	Amoxycyllin 250 mg b.d. Erythromycin 250 mg q.d.s. Doxycycline 100 mg o.d.	*Avoid* tetracycline, chloramphenicol Monitor liver function
Other infections as per organisms		
Tuberculosis	*First choice of treatment* Rifampicin 450–600 mg before breakfast INAH 5 mg/kg 3 times a week (post-dialysis) plus pyridoxine 20 mg daily plus Ethambutol 5 mg/kg o.d. plus dose at end of dialysis (for 8 weeks) or Pyrazinamide 20–35 mg/kg o.d. in 3–4 divided doses, for 8 weeks	Monitor visual field Monitor liver function
	Alternatives Streptomycin 0.5 g twice a week PAS 2 g post-dialysis Capreomycin 15–20 mg/kg at end of dialysis Ethionamide 500–750 mg o.d. at night Thiacetazone 100 mg o.d.	Ototoxic Gastro-intestinal irritation Ototoxic Gastro-intestinal effects, hepatotoxic, neurotoxic Gastro-intestinal irritation, hepatotoxic

Drugs and dialysis

A comprehensive list of the effects of both haemo- and peritoneal dialysis has been given by C.J. Richard (1981) *Dialysis and Transplantation* **10**; 471 and in *Drug Prescribing in Renal Failure* dosing guidelines for adults based on material published in the *American Journal of Kidney Diseases* (1983) 3: 155–193; COBE Lab. Inc. Lakewood Co. USA

12.4 Drug interactions

For details of drug interactions see Ivan Stockley, *Drug Interaction Alert 13* (1990) (Boehringer Ingelheim). Important drug interactions in patients with renal disease include those shown in Table 12.4.

12.5 Compounds known to have induced haemolysis of G6PD-deficient red cells

Analgesics	Nonsulphonamide antibacterial
Acetanilid	agents (*contd*)
Acetylsalicylic acid*	Nitrofurantoin (Furadantin)
Acetophenetidin (phenacetin)	Chloramphenicol
Antipyrine	(Chloromycetin)
Aminopyrine (Pyramidon)	*Para*-aminosalicylic acid
Sulphonamides and sulphones	**Miscellaneous**
Sulphanilamide	Naphthalene (moth balls)
Sulphapyridine	Vitamin K (water soluble
N_2 acetylsulphanilamide	analogues)
Sulphacetamide	Probenecid (Benemid)
Sulphisoxazole (Gentrisin)*	Trinitrotoluene
Thiazolsulphone	Methylene blue
(Promizole)	Dimercaprol (BAL)
Sulphoxone (Diasone)	Phenylhydrazine
Trimethroprim (Septrin)	Quinine†
Nonsulphonamide antibacterial	Quinidine†
agents	**Antimalarials**
Furazolidone (Furoxone)	Primaquine
	Pamaquine
	Pentaquine
	Quinacrine (Atabrine)*

* Slightly haemolytic in Blacks, only in very large doses
† Haemolytic in Caucasians, but not in Blacks

Table 12.4 Drug interactions.

Drugs	Consequence of interaction
Allopurinol + azathioprine	Marrow depression, especially with renal failure
Allopurinol + warfarin	Anticoagulation potentiated, especially with renal failure
Aminoglycosides + frusemide	Nephrotoxicity and ototoxicity
Antacids + doxycycline Iron + doxycycline	Absorption of doxycycline reduced
Corticosteroids + rifampicin	Steroid levels reduced (transplant rejection)
Corticosteroids + live vaccines	Generalized reactions
Frusemide + indomethacin	Diuretic effect reduced
Warfarin + { cimetidine, clofibrate, co-trimoxazole }	Anticoagulation potentiated
Warfarin + { corticosteroids, rifampicin }	Anticoagulation reduced
Cyclosporin + erythromycin, cimetidine + ranitidine, ketoconazole, danazol, methyltestosterone	Elevates cyclosporin levels
Cyclosporin + anticonvulsants, rifampicin, co-trimoxazole i.v.	Lowers cyclosporin levels
Cyclosporin + aminoglycosides, indomethacin, amphoteracin B	Increased nephrotoxicity

Appendix

A1 Calculation for body size

The body surface area (m^2)

$$= \sqrt{\frac{\text{Ht (cm)} \times \text{weight (kg)}}{3600}}$$

or

$$\sqrt{\frac{\text{Ht (inches)} \times \text{weight (lb)}}{3131}}$$

(Mosteller RD (1987) *New Eng J Med* **317**: 1098)

A2 Nomogram for phosphate threshold

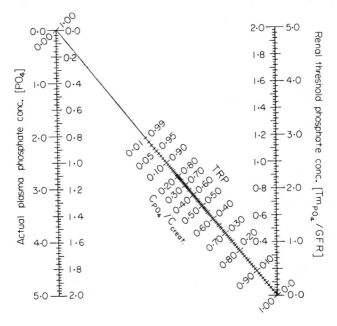

Fig. A1 Nomogram for phosphate threshold. (Reproduced from Walton RS and Bijvoet OLM (1975) Lancet, *ii:* 309.)

Procedure

A 2-hourly urine collection is obtained, together with a blood sample. The plasma and urinary creatinine and phosphate concentration levels are measured and the phosphate/creatinine clearance ratio, or fractional tubular reabsorbtion of phosphate (TRP), obtained from

$$\frac{CPO_4^{3-}}{C_{Cr}} = \frac{UPO_4^{3-}\ Cr}{U_{Cr}\ PO_4^{3-}}$$

and

$$TRP = 1 - \frac{CPO_4^{3-}}{C_{Cr}}$$

where UPO_4^{3-} is urinary phosphate, U_{Cr} urinary creatinine, PO_4^{3-} plasma phosphate, Cr plasma creatinine, C clearance, all in consistent units. The renal threshold phosphate concentration ($TmPO_4^{3-}/GFR$) can be derived by joining values of plasma phosphate levels and TRP (or CPO_4^{3-}/C_{Cr}). The units must correspond (i.e. they should be either S.I. or % mg).

The normal range is 0.8–1.35 mmol/l or 2.5–4.2 mg/100 ml in mass units. Patients with hyperparathyroidism usually have $TmPO_4^{3-}/GFR$ of <2.5 mg/dl and nearly always less than 2.7 mg/dl.

A3 Nomogram for gentamycin/tobramycin dosage

To determine a gentamicin/tobramycin dose schedule

Patient not receiving dialysis treatment
1 Join with a straight line the serum creatinine concentration appropriate to the sex on scale A and the age on scale B. Mark the point at which the straight line cuts line C.
2 Join with a straight line the mark on line C and the body weight on scale D. Mark the points at which this line cuts the dosage lines L and M.
3 The loading dose (mg) is written against the marked part of line L. The maintenance dose (mg) and the appropriate interval

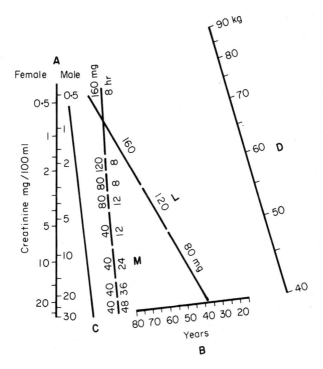

Fig. A2 Nomogram for gentamycin/tobramycin dosage.

(hours) between doses are written against the marked part of line M.

4 The nomogram is designed to give serum concentrations of gentamicin within the range 3–10 μg/ml 2 hours after each dose. In patients with renal insufficiency it is still desirable to perform check assays and to make appropriate dose adjustment.

5 To convert creatinine μmol/l to mg/100 ml, divide by 88.

Patient receiving dialysis treatment
Give 1 mg/kg i.m. at end of dialysis.

A4 Investigations

Water deprivation tests

Most healthy people have concentrated urine — a simple test is to measure the osmolality of an overnight sample of urine. If this exceeds 700 mmol/kg water, no further investigations are usually required since the hypothalamic-ADH-collecting duct axis is intact.

A more formal dehydration test is as follows. The patient is weighed and then deprived of all fluids. The weight should be measured every 3–4 hours and if 4% of the body weight is lost the test is terminated. Dehydration continues for up to 24 hours. The osmolality of at least one sample of urine passed between 12 and 24 hours should exceed 900 mmol/kg water.

Tests of urinary concentrating ability using pitressin

1 Pitressin tannate in oil is no longer available.
2 DDAVP (Desamino-cys-1-8-D arginine vasopressin), is a synthetic analogue of arginine vasopressin. 4 μg is given i.m. and aliquots of urines collected over 24 hours are measured for osmolality. In normal subjects the maximum urine osmolality should exceed 800 mmol/kg water.

Ammonium chloride test

Do not undertake if bicarbonate (Tco_2) < 20 mmol/l

Short test
1 Collect hourly samples of urine from 8–12 noon.
2 Take a sample of venous blood at 10.00 a.m. for electrolytes including bicarbonate.
3 Give 0.1 g of ammonium chloride/kg body weight in gelatine capsules orally at 12.00 noon, together with a litre of water, over about 1 hour.
4 Take a further blood sample at 2.00 p.m. for electrolytes and bicarbonate.

5 Urine samples are obtained at hourly intervals for 6 hours (12 noon–6.00 p.m.) during which the pH should fall below 5.3.

Long test
The control period is extended for 2–3 days and the administration of ammonium chloride is spread over 5 days, giving 7.5 g/day in divided doses. At the end of 4–5 days the pH should have fallen to below 5.0.

A5 Correction for calcium

Several equations have been given but the following has been recommended:

adjusted calcium (mmol/l) = measured calcium (mmol/l)
+ 0.02 (40-albumin (g/l)).

For example,
$$\text{measured calcium} = 1.85 \text{ mmol/l,}$$
$$\text{albumin} = 20 \text{ g/l,}$$
$$\text{then adjusted calcium} = 1.85 + (0.02 \times 20)$$
$$= 2.25 \text{ mmol/l (normal).}$$

A6 Diets

All dietetic advice should be obtained through a dietitian. The following tables give the composition of certain common foods:
● foods high in potassium—to be avoided
● foods high in sodium—to be avoided
● foods high in phosphorus
● foods high and low in oxalate

Foods high in potassium—to be avoided

Nuts—including peanuts, cashew nuts, coconut
Ice-cream, yoghurt, etc.
Chocolate and all chocolate products, including chocolate drinks
and cakes and biscuits
Instant coffee, instant tea, malted milk drinks

Molasses and black treacle
All beers, lagers and concentrated fruit drinks, e.g. Ribena,
    frozen and canned orange juice, cider
Fruit squashes and mineral waters
Dried fruits, e.g. dates, raisins, etc.
Salt substitutes, e.g. Ruthmol, Selora, etc.
Dried vegetables
Curry powder
Salt-free baking powder

Foods high in sodium — to be avoided

- do not use salt in the cooking
- do not add salt at the table

*Foods preserved or processed with salt and foods with a high
natural salt content*
Meats and fish or poultry that is tinned, smoked, cured or
pickled, e.g. bacon, ham, salt pork, salt beef, salt tongue, all
sausages, luncheon meat, corned beef, smoked fish, sardines,
kippers, etc.
Meat and fish pastes, canned meat stews, etc.
Shellfish — crab, lobster, shrimps, scallops
Dehydrated prepacked meals
Cheese
Tinned vegetables
Tinned and packet soups
Breakfast cereals

Salted relishes and seasonings
Chutney, commercial pickles, bottled sauces, e.g. brown sauce,
tomato sauce, salad cream
Prepared mustard and horseradish
Meat extracts, Marmite, Bovril, Oxo, Barmene
Gravy mixes

Salt substitutes and flavourings and other sodium compounds
Culinary salts, e.g. garlic salt, onion salt, celery salt
Monosodium glutamate, e.g. Aromat

Meat tenderizers
Baking powder, baking soda
Bicarbonate of soda, fruit salts, indigestion tablets

Self-raising flour and products
Commercial cakes, biscuits and scones and pastry, instant
pudding and cake mixes

Milk beverage flavourings
Horlicks, Ovaltine, Bournvita, chocolate, cocoa

Miscellaneous foods
Chocolate (all kinds)
Toffees, fudge, fruit gums
Nuts (all kinds)
Dried fruits, e.g. raisins, sultanas, currants, prunes and figs
Black treacle, syrup, peanut butter, meat and fish paste
Ice-cream, mousse
Evaporated and condensed milk
Potato crisps
Instant coffee
Coffee essence

Foods high in phosphorus—to be avoided

Meat, fish, cheese, eggs—other than in quantities given on
diet sheet
Condensed milk
Baking powder
Curry powder
All nuts except chestnuts and coconuts
Dried vegetables and fruit
Bournvita, cocoa powder, Horlicks, Nescafe, Ovaltine
All-Bran, Puffed Wheat, Shredded Wheat, Weetabix, Grapenuts
Allinson's bread, malt bread
Ryvita, Vita-wheat
Bemax, Farex
Chocolates, toffees, ice-cream

Relative oxalate content in some foods and beverages

High oxalate content

Rhubarb	Sweet potatoes	Tea
Spinach	Dill	Some instant coffee
Beet greens	Nuts	Grapefruit juice
Swiss chard	Unripe bananas	Orange juice
Turnip greens	Chocolate	Cranberry juice
Beets	Cocoa	Grape juice
Sorrell	Ovaltine	Pepper
Parsley		

Low oxalate content

Meats	Peas	Melons
Fish	Turnips	Peaches
Dairy products	Lettuce	Pears
Eggs	Radishes	Pineapple
Cereals	Apples	Plums
Cabbage	Ripe bananas	Raspberries
Asparagus	Apricots	Margarine
Cauliflower		

A7 Diagnosis of brain death

Department of Health and Social Security (1986) *Cadaveric Organs for Transplantation* Appendix 5 pp. 33–39

1 The patient is deeply comatose and the coma is not due to depressant drugs, hypothermia or any metabolic or endocrine cause.

2 The patient is being maintained on a ventilator because spontaneous respiration had previously become inadequate or had ceased altogether (exclude the effect of muscle relaxants).

3 There should be no doubt that the patient's condition is due to irremediable structural brain damage. The diagnosis of a disorder which can lead to brain death should have been fully established.

Diagnostic tests for the confirmation of brain death

All brainstem reflexes are absent:
- fixed pupils unresponsive to light
- lack of corneal reflux
- absent vestibular-ocular reflexes
- no motor responses within the cranial nerve distribution can be elicited by adequate stimulation of any somatic area
- there is no gag reflex or response to bronchial stimulation
- no respiratory movements occur when the ventilator is disconnected and the $P\text{CO}_2$ rises to 50 mmHg

Other considerations

- the tests should be repeated, at least once, the time interval being determined by the clinical state
- spinal cord reflexes may be left intact in brain-dead patients
- EEG confirmation is not necessary for the diagnosis of brain death
- the body temperature should be above 35°C
- specialist opinion should be that of a consultant or his deputy (who should have been registered 5 years or more and have had adequate experience in such cases) and 'one other doctor' — whom many believe should be an experienced neurologist

A8   Normal concentration ranges

Plasma	SI units	Traditional units
Sodium	135−145 mmol/l	135−145 mEq/l
Potassium	3.5−5.0 mmol	3.5−5.0 mEq/l
Chloride	95−105 mmol/l	95−105 mEq/l
Bicarbonate	24−30 mmol/l	24−30 mEq/l
Urea	2.5−6.5 mmol/l	15−40 mg/dl
Creatinine	42−130 μmol/l	0.4−1.5 mg/dl
Uric acid	0.12−0.42 mmol/l	3.0−7.0 mg/dl
Lactate	0.6−1.8 mmol/l	0.6−1.8 mg/dl
Lithium	< 2.0 mmol/l	< 2.0 mEq/l
Osmolality	285−295 mmol/kg water	285−295 mosm/kg water
Renin	1.7−2.1 pmol/ml/h	Recumbent, depends
Aldosterone	150−450 pmol/l	on sodium intake

24 hour urine	SI units	Traditional units
Creatinine clearance	1.7−2.1 ml/s/1.73 m^2	
Protein	< 150 mg	< 150 mg
Calcium	< 7.5 mmol	< 300 mg
Urate	<3.8 mmol (women)	<700 mg (women)
	<4.4 mmol (men)	<800 mg (men)
Oxalate	0.1−0.46 mmol	15−50 mg
Cystine	−	10−100 mg
β$_2$ microglobulin	−	4−370 μg/l
	−	30−370 μg/24 hour

Serum	SI units	Traditional units
Calcium	2.2−2.6 mmol/l	8.8−10.4 mg/dl
Ionized calcium	1.12−1.47 mmol/l	4.5−5.9 mg/dl
Magnesium	0.7−1.0 mmol/l	1.4−2.0 mEq/l
Phosphate	0.75−1.35 mmol/l	3.0−5.40 mg/dl
Albumin	35−45 g/l	3.5−5.0 g/dl
Globulin	19−23 g/l	2.3−3.5 g/dl
Aluminium	< 3 μmol/l	< 80 μg/dl
IgG	5.5−14.5 g/l	540−1450 mg/dl
IgA	0.5−32 g/l	50−320 mg/dl
IgM	0.5−3.1 g/l	50−310 mg/dl
C3	0.8−1.8 g/l	80−180 mg/dl
C4	0.13−0.43 g/l	13−43 mg/dl
Bilirubin	5−17 μmol/l	0.4−1.0 mg/dl
Alkaline phosphatase	90−250 u/l	3−13 King Armstrong u/l
ALT	0.08−0.32 μmol/s/l	< 35 iu/l
AST	0.08−0.32 μmol/s/l	< 30 iu/l
CPK	0.08−0.58 μmol/s/l	5−50 iu/l
Cholesterol	3.4−6.5 mmol/l	130−250 mg/dl
Triglycerides	0.5−2.2 mmol/l	25−150 mg/dl
Ferritin	20−200 μg/l	20−200 ng/ml
PTH (terminal)	< 0.5 μg/l	−
25-OH vitamin D_3	15−100 nmol/l	−
β_2 microglubulin	−	1.1−2.4 mg/l

CPK: creatinine phosphokinase; ALT: alanine aminotranferase; and AST: aspartate aminotransferase

List of abbreviations

ACTH	Adrenocorticotrophic hormone
ADH	Antidiuretic hormone
AFB	Acid-fast bacillus
AHA	Acetohydroxamic acid
ALG	Antilymphocyte globulin
ALT	Alanine aminotranferase
ANF	Antinuclear factor
ARF	Acute renal failure
ASO	Antistreptolysin O titre
AST	Aspartate aminotransferase
ATG	Antithymocyte globulin
A-V	Arterio-venous
b.d.	Twice daily
BP	Blood pressure
CAPD	Continuous ambulatory peritoneal dialysis
CAVH	Continuous artero-venous haemofiltration
CAVHD	Continuous artero-venous haemodialysis
CMV	Cytomegalovirus
COLA	Cystine, ornithine, lysine and arginine
CPK	Creatinine phosphokinase
CSF	Cerebrospinal fluid
CSU	Catheter sample of urine
CVP	Central venous pressure
CVVHD	Continuous veno-venous haemodialysis
CXR	Chest X-ray
DMSO	Dimethylsulphoxide
DMSA	Dimercaptosuccinic acid
DTPA	Di-ethylenetriamine penta-acetic acid
ECF	Extracellular fluid
ECG	Electrocardiogram

EDTA	Ethylenediaminetetra-acetic acid
EEG	Electroencephalogram
EMU	Early morning urine
ESR	Erythrocyte sedimentation rate
FBC	Full blood count
FMF	Familial Mediterranean fever
GBM	Glomerular basement membrane
GFR	Glomerular filtration rate
GN	Glomerulonephritis
G6PD	Glucose-6-phosphate-dehydrogenase
HGPT	Hypoxanthine-guanine phosphoribosyl transferase
i.m.	Intramuscular
i.v.	Intravenous
IVU	Intravenous urogram
JVP	Jugular venous pressure
KCCT	Kaolin cephalin clotting time
LH	Luteinising hormone
MIC	Minimal inhibitory concentration
MLC	Mixed lymphocyte culture
MRC	Medical Research Council
MSU	Midstream specimen of urine
N saline	Normal saline, with a concentration of Na^+, 150 mmol/l and Cl^-, 150 mmol/l
NAG	N-acetyl-β-D-glucosaminidase
NSU	Non-specific urethritis
o.d.	Once a day
PAH	*Para*-aminohippuric acid

PCV	Packed cell volume
PRA	Plasma renin activity
PTH	Parathyroid hormone
PUO	Pyrexia of unknown origin
q.d.s	Four times daily
RA	Rheumatoid arthritis
RBC	Red blood cell count
RPF	Renal plasma flow
RTA	Renal tubular acidosis
SLE	Systemic lupus erythematosus
SPA	Suprapubic aspiration urine sample
$T_{1/2}$	Half life
t.d.s	Thrice daily
Tm	Maximal tubular reabsorption
TRH	Thyroid-releasing hormone
TRP	Tubular reabsorption of phosphate
TSH	Thyroid-stimulating hormone
VMA	Vanilmandelic acid

Further reading

New topics in nephrology are being introduced constantly and this requires assiduous reading of journals. Textbooks which the author has found particularly useful include the following.

General textbooks

Schrier RW and Gottschalk CW (1988) *Diseases of the Kidney.* Little, Brown and Company, Boston.
This is a large, comprehensive textbook.
de Wardener HE (1985) *The Kidney, an Outline of Normal Structure and Function.* Churchill Livingstone, Edinburgh.
This is a readable, physiologically orientated smaller textbook.

Specialized topics

Crawfurd MD'A (1988) *The Genetics of Renal Tract Disorders.* Oxford University Press, Oxford.
A detailed review of the genetics of renal diseases.
Coe FL (1988) *Nephrolithiasis.* Chicago Year Book Publication, Chicago.
Holliday MA, Barratt TM and Vernier RL (1987) *Paediatric Nephrology.* Williams and Wilkins, Baltimore.
Kunin CM (1987) *Detection, Prevention and Management of Urinary Tract Infections.* Lea and Febiger, Philadelphia.
A classic book on management of urinary tract infections.
Morris PJ (ed) (1988) *Kidney Transplantation. Principles and Practice.* WB Saunders, London.
A comprehensive review of transplantation.
Schrier RW (1986) *Renal and Electrolyte Disorders.* Little, Brown and Company, Boston.
A well-written physiological but practical textbook.

Index

Page numbers in *italics* indicate figures, and in **bold** indicate tables